RECHARGING YOUR LIFE
WITH PEMF THERAPY

Empower Your Natural Healing Potential

I0039474

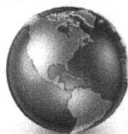

GLOBAL
PUBLISHING
G R O U P

Global Publishing Group
Australia • New Zealand • Singapore • America • London

RECHARGING YOUR LIFE
WITH PEMF THERAPY

Empower Your Natural Healing Potential

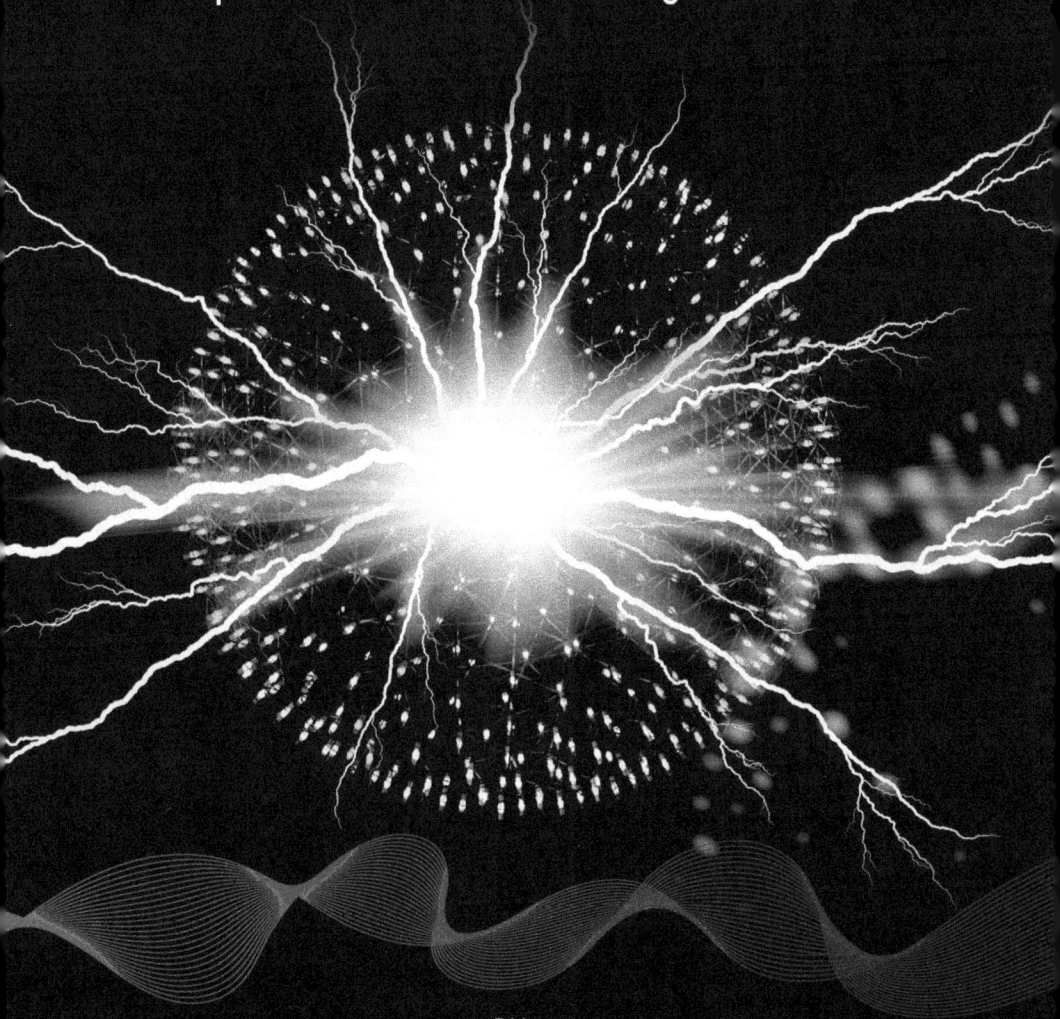

BY
GARY WOOLUMS

DISCLAIMER

The information and advice contained in or made available throughout this book is for informational and educational purposes only. It is not intended to replace or substitute the advice and/or services of a physician or any other healthcare professional. There is no intention to prescribe or make specific health claims for any of the technologies or products mentioned in the book. Any attempt to diagnose and treat illness should come under the direction and supervision of a licensed health care practitioner. Consult with a physician in all matters relating to health, particularly with respect to any symptoms that may require further diagnosis or medical attention.

Any products mentioned in the book are not intended for use in the diagnosis of disease or other conditions, or in the cure, mitigation, treatment or prevention of disease in humans or animals. PEMF therapy does not cure anything. PEMF therapy boosts cellular voltage potential. This can increase the biological efficiency of the body, which may help to restore or maintain health.

The information contained in this book is for general information purposes only. While the information provided is intended to be up to date and correct, I make no representations or warranties of any kind, express or implied, about the completeness, accuracy, reliability, suitability or availability with respect to the information, products, services or related graphics contained in the book for any purpose. Any reliance placed on such information is therefore strictly at your own risk.

National Library of Australia
Cataloguing-in-Publication entry:

Recharging Your Life With PEMF Therapy: Empower Your Natural Healing Potential - Gary Woolums

1st ed.
ISBN: 978-1-925370-88-1 (pbk.)

A catalogue record for this book is available from the National Library of Australia

Published by Global Publishing Group
PO Box 258, Banyo, QLD 4014 Australia
Email admin@globalpublishinggroup.com.au

For further information about orders:
Phone: +61 7 3267 0747

DEDICATION

This book is dedicated to the elemental energy of Nature and the balancing energy of femininity through which all is born and created. In my world, 80% of those who are pulled to and resonate with PEMF therapy are women. I'm blessed to be a part of a journey of learning that has led to feeling so much gratitude for the healing and nurturing energy of feminine energy. We live in a time and global ethos that is severely devoid of the balance and nourishing spirit of femininity, which is central and fundamental to the foundation of life and Nature. Most importantly, I'm *very* blessed that Lisbeth has graced my life with her unique beauty, positivity and her ever *presence in the moment* that manifests on so many levels. And now my life has a new and special element of Grace. I am so blessed!

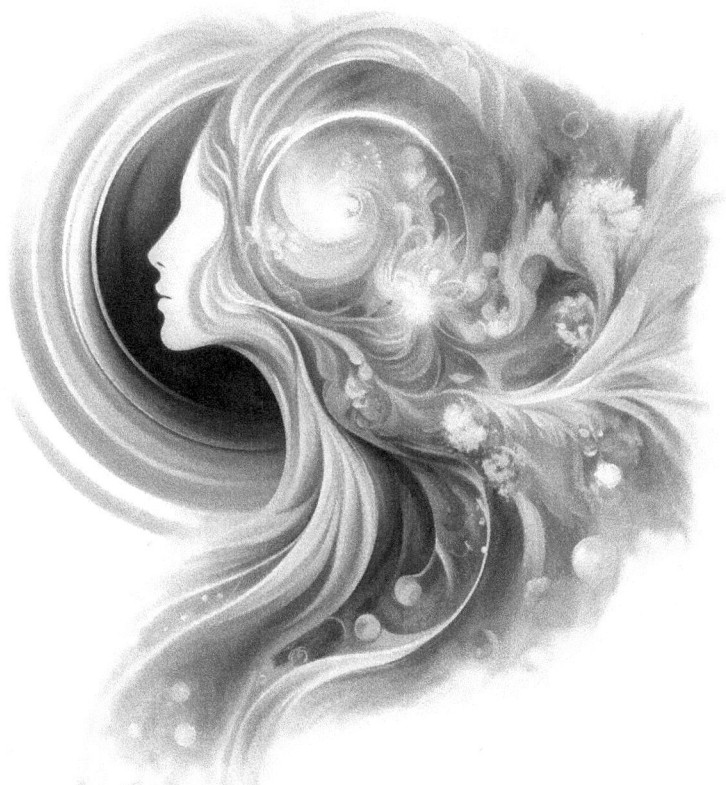

CONTENTS

INTRODUCTION

"The greatest obstacle to discovery is not ignorance; it is the illusion of knowledge."
– Daniel J. Boorstin

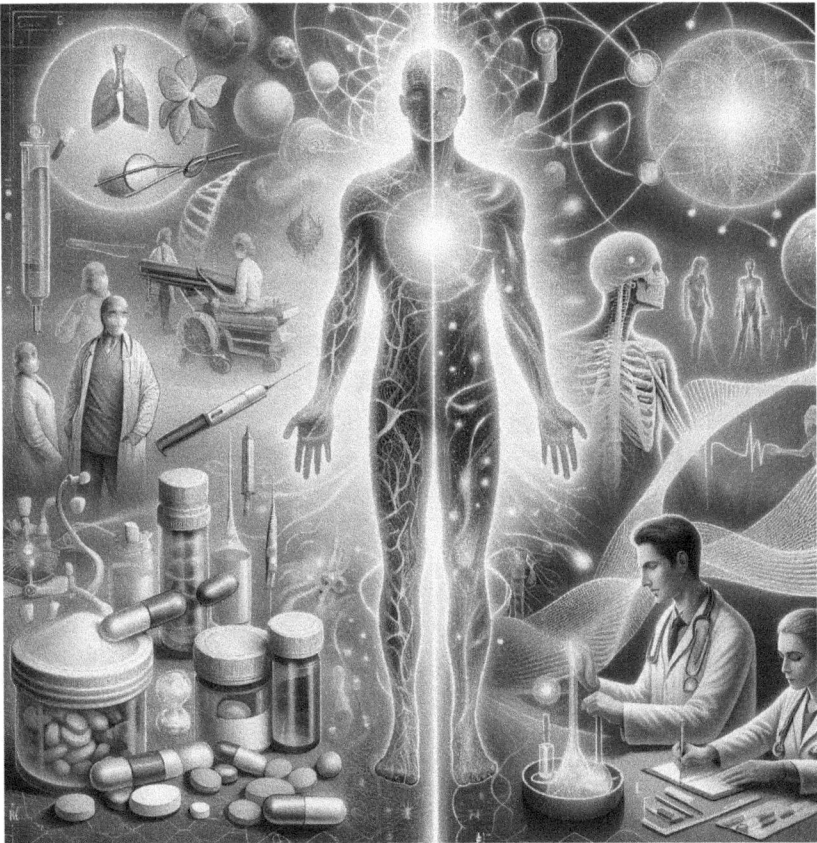

I begin with this quote because it resonates on several levels. I'm addressing the reluctance of conventional Western medicine to integrate biophysics into its narrowly focused molecular biology framework. Biophysics is the field that applies the theories and methods of physics to understand how the bioelectrical systems work in the body. Physics is the energy of everything on many levels. Conventional medicine measures the electrical activity of the heart and the brain but doesn't investigate the bioelectrical potentials for healing. The human body is far more than just a biochemical organism to be dispensed pharmaceuticals or cut open to remove diseased tissue. Physics, or in this case – biophysics, addresses one of the most fundamental levels on which all cells and systems communicate and are governed within the body. Its time is now.

Writing this book has been a challenge to balance my opinions and experience regarding PEMF therapy along with the current scientific theories put into practice on a daily basis. This book is written to educate people about PEMF at a basic level. I know it doesn't come close to explaining all the intricacies of communication that transpire at the cellular level. Hopefully more scientists will follow the work of Michael Levin, Richard Nuccitelli, James Oschman and all those before that have pioneered research into the biophysics of the body. It's a field that is constantly evolving and changing as new technology and discoveries slowly slip through the cracks of the dogmatic mindset of most of the scientific and medical community.

The Purpose of this Book

I wrote this book for several reasons:

The first is to educate people who want to learn more about PEMF therapy in regard to how it works and whether it may be able to help them or a loved one. I know my explanations may not adequately describe the intricate complexities that actually come into play when PEMF is applied within the body. I've aimed to keep it simple, but at times, simplicity can't fully encompass all the essential points that need to be addressed or are still unknown.

The second reason for this book is to show how this proven technology can be highly beneficial in the wellness industry. This technology can be adopted to boost the beneficial outcomes of an existing healthcare practice of any kind or a completely new business on its own. I don't know one practitioner who has added PEMF to their practice that is not amazed by some of the outcomes they've seen. PEMF has significantly increased the potential to help people and it also broadens the range of the health issues that can be treated. Besides healthcare workers, PEMF has taken up residence in gyms, aged care facilities, wellness centers, corporate wellness programs, hair/beauty salons and mental health practices to name a few examples.

I am not aware of any current technology that comes close to doing what PEMF therapy can do to help so many people with so many different kinds of health-related issues in such an easy, safe and noninvasive way. PEMF is supported by peer-reviewed clinical studies conducted over several decades, demonstrating a variety of health benefits. The last count I saw was over one hundred and fifty.

"PEMF is the crown jewel of energy medicine."
- Bryant Meyers, physicist, author and 25-year researcher on energy medicine.

If you had seen what I've seen PEMF therapy can do for people and understand the basic principles of how it works, then you would purchase a system *right now*, even if there's nothing wrong with you and do it every day for the rest of your life. Read on and I'll tell you why.

My Experience with PEMF

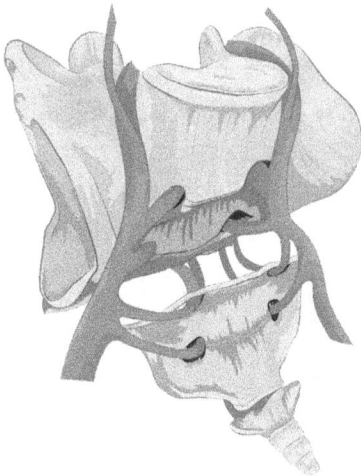

In 1989, I was in a very serious accident where I broke my back. My sacrum, the large triangular-shaped bone at the base of my spine, was sheared completely in two. The lower detached bone was moved completely out of alignment with my spine. The orthopedic specialists said there was nothing that could be done. It was too risky to operate because the major sacral nerves and blood vessels pass through four large openings on each side of the sacrum.

I ended up on crutches for seven months. While the major pain subsided after about nine months, I was still left with chronic pain, inflammation and stiffness that waxed and waned in varying degrees over the years. It was always there and I thought it always would be. I tried every complementary or alternative therapy I could find using

Introduction

at least forty to fifty different health practitioners over the years. I got symptomatic relief some of the time, but it didn't last. I spent over fifty thousand dollars during those twenty-six years. I was seeing someone about my back at least once every two weeks. I could have easily gone twice a week for symptomatic relief, if I could have afforded it.

In 2017 after two or three months of research about PEMF, I had to purchase a system because I couldn't find anyone that offered treatments in my area. I only found one person online in all of Australia for that matter. Once I received my system, I did a treatment twice a day on the full-body mat and the smaller pad for a half hour each time. At the end of the first week the symptoms were 80% gone. In around two weeks, most of the symptoms had disappeared.

The key point is that the pain has not returned for over seven years up to the time of this writing. To top that, I now sleep about one to one and a half hours less and don't get up in the middle of the night nearly as often. Also, when I wake up, I feel much more refreshed and fully awake. I simply have more energy. There's no sleep inertia like there used to be where it took me awhile to wake up. I still use PEMF twice a day for about a half hour each time and will for the rest of my life.

CHAPTER 1
What is PEMF Therapy?

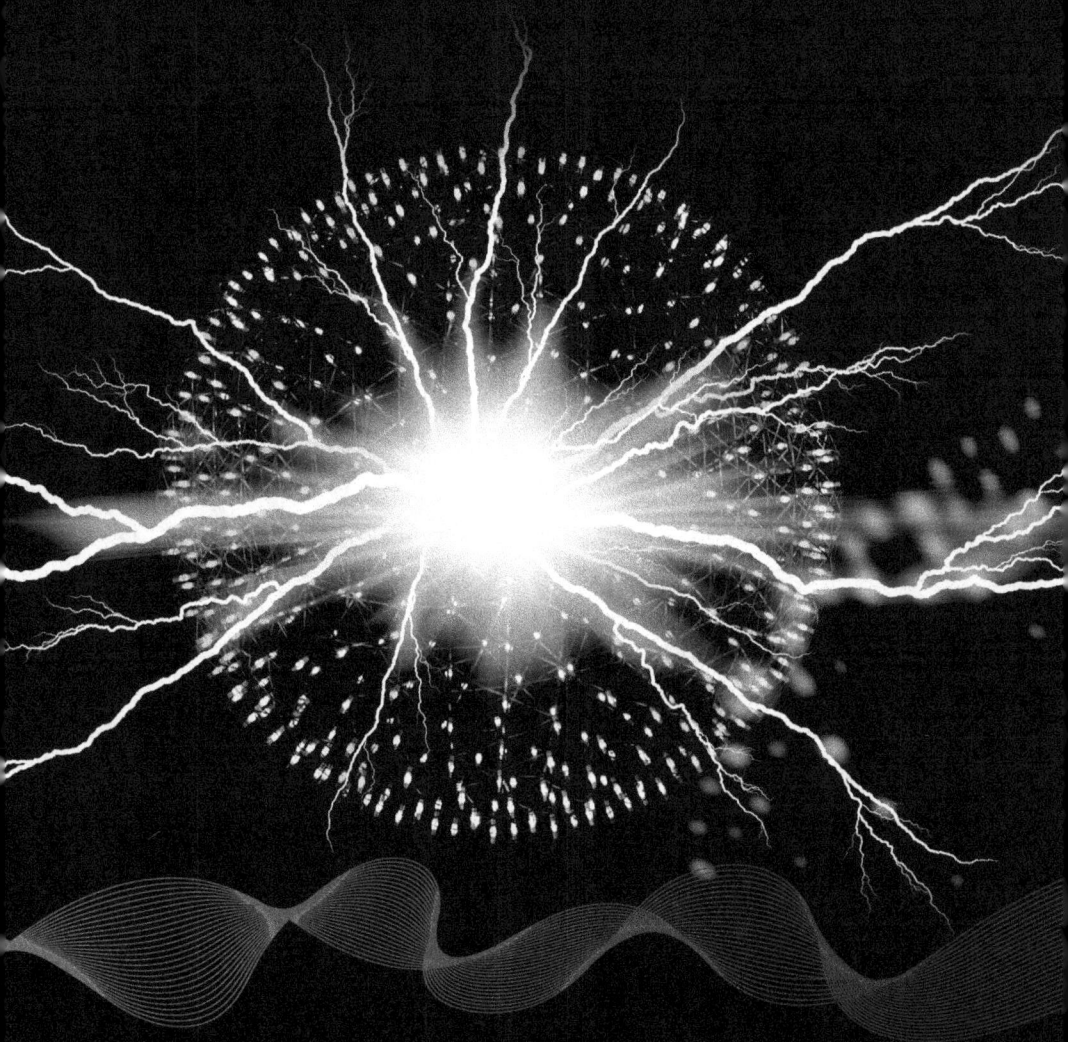

CHAPTER 1
What is PEMF Therapy?

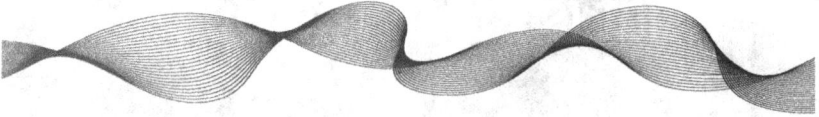

The Potential of PEMF Therapy

In the dynamic tapestry of technical medical advancements, one natural thread stands out for its potential to weave together the realms of science and natural therapy in a safe and noninvasive way. Pulsed Electromagnetic Field (PEMF) therapy, once on the fringes of Western medicine, has emerged as a significant force in the quest for a clinically proven treatment that delivers results.

PEMF's potential extends across a broad spectrum of ailments from chronic pain to neurological disorders, from accelerated recovery to enhanced athletic performance and from mental imbalance to sleep improvement. What's more, PEMF is backed by thousands of clinical studies showing a multitude of benefits. Yet, relatively speaking, very few people in the health professions or the general public know about PEMF.

The potential of PEMF therapy extends beyond the confines of clinic studies or the laboratory. It speaks to a fundamental truth about the interconnectedness of all living things—a truth that resonates with ancient wisdoms and modern science alike. At its core, PEMF therapy reminds us that we are not separate from nature but intricately woven into the frequencies and the fields of its fabric, subject to its subtle rhythms and energies. PEMF, if applied with the resonating frequencies and intensities of Nature, amplifies the body's innate ability to heal by enhancing or energizing the bioelectrical systems within the body.

"Bioelectricity is the spark of life."
– Dr Michael Levin

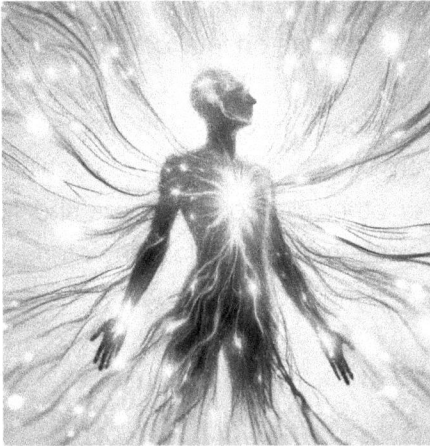

PEMF therapy is not a panacea or a cure-all, but rather a doorway to safe and effective possibilities in healthcare—a doorway that invites us to step beyond the confines and limitations of conventional thinking and into a world where healing and rejuvenation is not just a destination but a natural journey of self-discovery and empowerment.

PEMF (Pulsed Electromagnetic Field) therapy is a form of therapy that involves the use of electromagnetic fields to improve overall health and well-being. While thousands of studies have shown potential benefits, it's important to first be aware of the contraindications or precautions associated with PEMF therapy. It's also important to note that the scientific evidence and clinical studies supporting the effectiveness of PEMF therapy are still not readily accepted and therefore incorporated in the practice of Western Medicine. Nevertheless, PEMF therapy is slowly making inroads within some mainstream medical and scientific communities, especially in Europe and the US. I advise people to be sure to discuss *any* treatment, whether PEMF or any other alternative treatment, with their trusted healthcare professional. Many doctors may never have heard of it, but that is progressively changing.

Contraindications and Precautions for PEMF therapy include:

1. **Pregnancy:** Pregnant women are advised to avoid PEMF therapy, especially in the abdominal and pelvic regions, as there is limited research on its effects on fetal development.

2. **Implanted electronic devices:** People with implanted devices such as pacemakers, defibrillators, cochlear implants, insulin pumps or other electronic devices should avoid PEMF therapy. The electromagnetic fields may interfere with the proper functioning of these devices.

3. **Epilepsy** and seizure disorders: There is some concern that PEMF therapy may trigger seizures in individuals with epilepsy or a history of seizure disorders.

4. **Active bleeding:** Individuals with active bleeding, hemophilia or hemorrhagic conditions should avoid PEMF therapy, as it may potentially increase blood flow and exacerbate bleeding.

5. **Organ transplants:** People with recent organ transplants or who are on immunosuppressive medications should consult their healthcare provider before undergoing PEMF therapy, as there is a risk of PEMF stimulating the effectiveness of the immune system.

6. **PEMF** should only be used with the approval of a licensed health care professional for someone under medical supervision with the following conditions:

    - Presence of tumors
    - Serious cardiac arrhythmia
    - Acute attacks of hyperthyroidism
    - Extreme sensitivity to electromagnetic radiation

It's crucial to emphasize that the safety and efficacy of PEMF therapy are still areas of active research. Individuals considering this therapy should consult with their healthcare provider, especially if they have pre-existing medical conditions or concerns. Additionally, individuals should be wary of unsubstantiated claims from manufacturers or marketers of *any* PEMF system and therefore seek evidence-based information.

The Legitimacy of Energy Medicine & PEMF

Energy medicine is thought of as a relatively new science, but it has ancient origins in many different cultures where it was used and accepted for thousands of years in some cultures. Today, energy medicine can encompass many facets whether it's using the relatively new technology of PEMF or the old traditional and proven ways such as acupuncture, Reiki, Qi Gong, homeopathy, healing touch, etc.

Energy medicine is fundamentally based on the principles, dynamics and laws of physics, which Western medicine is steadfastly reluctant to incorporate within its science. Instead, conventional medicine takes the myopic approach that everything in the body is controlled by biochemistry and therefore predominately focuses on the use and many times abuse of pharmaceuticals. Thus, almost all research has been directed toward understanding the mechanisms of the chemistry of the body. This is done in order to be able to alter the biochemistry to alleviate the symptoms of disease. However, many biological dynamics cannot be sufficiently explained through biochemistry alone such as the electromagnetic fields and electrical currents within the body.

All of biology and biochemistry are governed by the principal laws of physics. Fundamentally, physics is the study of how energy works. Like all things, the human body is made up of and runs on energy or 'electrons,' if you don't like the word 'energy.' When the natural flow of energy (electrons) is blocked, disrupted or depleted, then the body becomes imbalanced. The body becomes bioelectrically and biochemically inefficient, which can contribute to many physiological disorders and imbalances.

Physics does not override the importance of the interactions of the biochemistry in the body. It's the principles or laws of physics that drives or governs much of the physiology of the body. It's very comparable to the system software of a computer.

'Electromagnetic energy is fundamental and the foundation of biology and medicine.'

– Dr James Oschman – "Energy Medicine, The Scientific Basis"

In 1989, the International Society for the Study of Subtle Energy and Energy Medicine was founded. Its aim is to study the informational systems and energies that interact with the human psyche and physiology, either enhancing or disrupting healthy equilibrium.

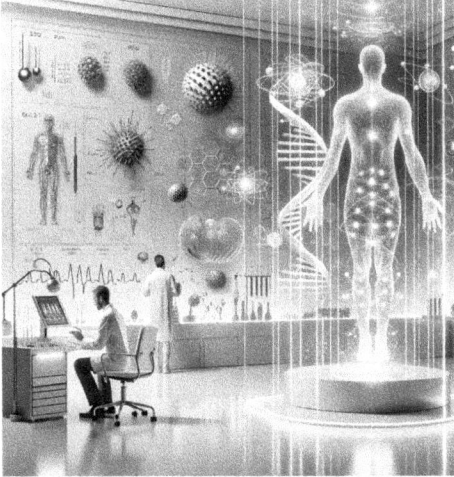

In the USA, energy medicine was put under official government guidelines in 1992, when the National Institutes of Health (NIH) established the National Center for Complementary and Alternative Medicine.

Even though energy medicine has been given *some* credibility by an official government health organization, that doesn't mean it has become readily accepted or adopted by Western Medicine. This is especially evident in the English-speaking countries where the government health organizations, which are supposed to protect people's lives have now become controlled agencies that protect the profits of corporations like pharmaceutical and pesticide manufacturers with total disregard for the consequences and loss of human life.

In Europe, especially in Eastern Europe, PEMF has been used in hospitals for years and also prescribed by doctors for over twenty years. Many well-known athletes have been quietly using PEMF for years to legally enhance their performance and to recover from competitions or injuries quicker. The horse racing industry readily adopted PEMF years ago because horses run faster and recover much quicker using PEMF.

PEMF therapy is currently used in the following fields:

1 – Alternative and Complementary Health: chiropractors, homeopaths, physiotherapists, naturopaths, nutritionists, massage therapists and many other related health professionals have added PEMF therapy to their practice. This has accomplished two things:

A – it's enhanced the effectiveness of their existing treatment modalities

B – it's expanded the spectrum of disorders they can effectively treat

As an example: A massage therapist with a PEMF system can help people with PTSD, sleep problems, stress & anxiety and autoimmune issues to name a few.

2 - Orthopedics and Sports Medicine: PEMF therapy is becoming widely accepted in orthopedics and sports medicine for treating musculoskeletal conditions, stimulating bone growth, reducing inflammation and alleviating pain.

3 - Pain Management: Some clinicians have incorporated PEMF therapy into effective pain management protocols. It is employed to manage chronic pain conditions, such as fibromyalgia and lower back pain.

4 - Wound Healing: In certain cases, PEMF therapy has shown benefits in wound healing.

5 - Neurology: There is ongoing research into the potential use of PEMF therapy in neurology, particularly for conditions such as depression, migraines, tinnitus and concussions.

6 – Cardiology: In some hospitals PEMF is used to help heal the massive chest wound after open heart surgery.

7 – Urology: PEMF is used to stimulate pelvic floor muscles, which designed to address pelvic floor dysfunction that can contribute to issues such as urinary incontinence.

8 - Plastic Surgery: PEMF is employed to stimulate microcirculation and cellular regeneration therefore bruising disappears much faster.

9 - Veterinary Medicine: PEMF therapy is more commonly used in veterinary medicine for conditions such as arthritis and post-surgical recovery in animals. It's extensively used by veterinarians or equine technicians involved in the horse racing industry and horses in general.

10 – Sports: PEMF is used in the field of sports on all levels for its potential benefits in various aspects of performance enhancement, injury management, rehabilitation, post-match recovery and injury prevention.

Awareness of PEMF therapy has significantly increased during my years of practice, particularly throughout the Covid period. Despite its niche within the broader field of complementary medicine, I'm still surprised by how many practitioners in the alternative health sector are unfamiliar with it. Among the general population, PEMF therapy remains relatively unknown but it is definitely changing.

Herein lies the opportunity for anyone who wants to get involved in a proven and easily administered technology, which has the potential to help many people with many different kinds of disorders in a safe and non-invasive way.

The Nature of Electromagnetic Fields

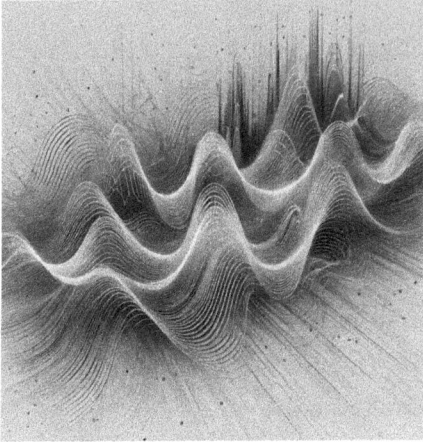

Electromagnetism is one of the four fundamental forces or energies of Nature. Electromagnetic fields include both electricity and magnetism. They are intrinsically intertwined; a moving electric current produces a magnetic field and changing magnetic field induces an electric current. The nature of the electromagnetic field is such that it can propagate through space in the form of waves. These waves carry energy and also information. They include radio waves, microwaves, infrared radiation, visible light, ultraviolet radiation, X-rays and gamma rays.

PEMF vs EMF

There's lots of debate about EMFs (electromagnetic fields) these days and their potential negative side-effects. I believe that EMFs are disruptive and have significant negative effects on health in spite of all of the official government and health organization denials. They have been doing the same denials for years regarding electric high power lines. They did it with DDT in the 50s, glyphosate now and the list goes on with Wi-Fi, cell or mobile phones and all the communication towers radiating EMFs everywhere. For me, it didn't take very many people coming to my practice reporting health disruptions of various kinds to make an association with EMFs. The most common correlation I see is when a new phone tower goes up in a neighborhood. People report that it is disruptive in many different ways, especially sleep, anxiety and brain fog. It is becoming more and more of a problem and has been labeled EHS (electromagnetic hypersensitivity).

"If you could eliminate certain outside frequencies that interfered in our bodies, we would have greater resistance toward disease."
– Nicola Tesla

PEMF (Pulsed Electromagnetic Field) and EMFs (Electromagnetic Fields) are related but distinct and separate elements in the electromagnetic spectrum.

PEMF: Pulsed Electromagnetic Field therapy refers to the therapeutic application of pulsating electromagnetic fields to the body for various health purposes. In my practice, the PEMFs are low frequency within the biological window of resonance and low intensity. In other words, they align with the natural magnetic field of the Earth. They are all based around the frequencies and intensities found within Nature, which also happen to correspond to the same frequencies we find within the human body.

EMFs: Electromagnetic Fields, on the other hand, encompass a much broader spectrum or much broader range of electromagnetic frequencies and intensities generated by many types of technology. This includes artificial sources (such as power lines, electronic devices and wireless communication systems like Wi-Fi, Bluetooth or cell/mobile phones, which have very, very high frequencies millions of time higher than PEMFs.

The health effects of EMFs are a subject of scientific investigation and rigorous debate. While some studies suggest possible associations between long-term exposure to certain EMFs and health risks, such as increased cancer risk or effects on sleep patterns, the evidence is mixed and further research is being advised. That's the 'official story line' on EMFS, but it's interesting to note that countries like Switzerland, Italy, France, Austria, Luxembourg, Bulgaria, Poland, Hungary, Israel, Russia and China have set exposure time limits for Wi-Fi in schools or they are completely banned. The use of smart phones in school is also being regulated in many countries.

Does it seem plausible to you that the constant influx of frequencies in the millions and billions of cycles per second, entering your brain, could be a factor in current or future health issues? The human brain operates at relatively low frequencies from .1 Hz (cycles per second) up to approximately 100 Hz. That's something to think about, especially if you or your kids have Bluetooth earbuds in the ears all day. That's 2.4 BILLION cycles a second radiating into the ears right next to your brain. To me, that doesn't feel right on any level and significantly fails if any kind of common sense is applied.

In summary, PEMF therapy is a specific therapeutic application that utilizes electromagnetic fields in a very narrow range for potential health benefits. EMFs encompass a much broader spectrum of electromagnetic fields, which have a broad range of intensities and frequencies along with arguably potential negative side effects.

PEMF vs Grounding (Earthing)

Many people over the years have asked me if PEMF is the same as grounding. Grounding refers to the direct connection or contact of the body to the Earth. It involves direct physical contact with the ground, such as walking barefoot on the beach, in the water, on grass or using grounding mats or conductive systems connected to the Earth by a wire. The purpose of grounding is to allow the transfer of electrical energy (electrons) between the Earth and the person. This potentially affects various physiological processes and promotes a sense of well-being. It's often associated with the idea of reconnecting with the Earth's natural electrical charge.

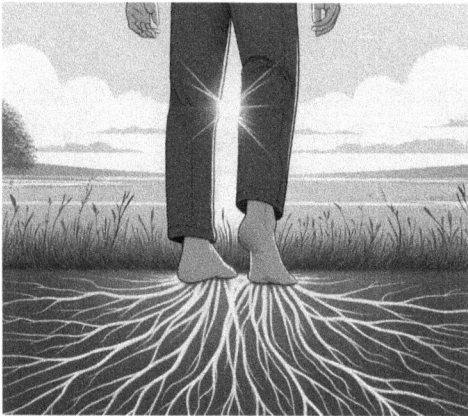

Grounding involves establishing a physical connection between the human body (or an object) and the Earth. This connection allows for the exchange of electrical energy between the Earth and the body. Here are some key points:

1. Direct Contact with the Earth:

- Grounding typically occurs through direct skin contact with the Earth's surface. This could involve activities like walking barefoot on soil, grass, sand or even swimming in natural bodies of water.

2. Electron Transfer:

- The Earth carries a natural, negative electrical charge. When a person makes direct contact with the Earth, electrons from the Earth flow into the body if there is a lesser charge in the body. Electrons are negatively charged particles, and this transfer of electrons can neutralize excess positive charges (free radicals) within the body.

3. Potential Health Benefits:

- Proponents of grounding suggest that this electron transfer has various health benefits. This includes reducing inflammation, improving sleep, normalizing cortisol levels (related to stress), and promoting a general sense of well-being.

4. Connection to Nature:

- Grounding is often seen as a way to reconnect with nature in our modern, urbanized lifestyles. Advocates say that spending time outdoors and establishing a connection with the Earth's natural energy can have positive effects on health and vitality.

5. Grounding Products:

- Some people use grounding products, such as conductive mats or sheets, which are connected to the Earth through the electrical grounding system in homes. These products aim to simulate the effects of direct contact with the Earth, allowing individuals to experience grounding benefits indoors.

In the past, I used a grounding system on my bed and I also tried a grounding mat that I used at my desk for approximately nine months. It was at the time when I had already adopted PEMF and was using it twice a day and everyday (still do). I didn't notice any significant difference after adding grounding to the equation.

That's not to say I don't think there are any benefits. I've heard many reports from people saying that grounding has helped in regard to most of the benefits listed above. I'd advise not to purchase the sheets for a bed because the conducive strands will break after time due to wear and tear. Plus, a washing machine can damage the conductive strands. This advice was given to me by a manufacturer of the sheets. I purchased their mattress pad that lays under the sheet. It's not as good as the direct connection with a sheet, but will last much longer.

Charging Water with PEMF

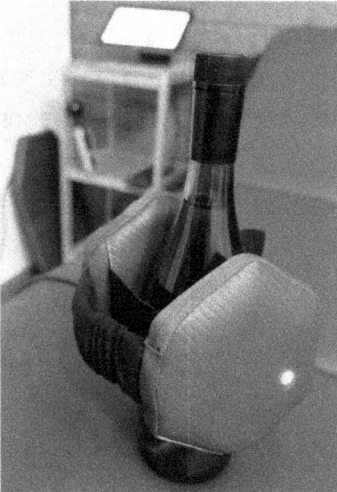

One of the very unique things you can do with PEMF is to charge water. You do this by filling a glass container with filtered water and place the container over one of the coils on the mat or the pad. I personally use a glass wine bottle and like to charge three or four bottles each day and try to drink as much of the charged water as I can. I charge them for thirty minutes at the earth's natural intensity.

Don't use a metal container and don't use a glass container with a metal cap. Preferably don't use a plastic container. The restructuring or charging of the water does not last all day. The molecular bond angles revert back to their normal state within eight to twelve hours. So, the water is good for a day.

Water that is treated with PEMF has some unique properties. The first thing people notice is that it literally feels different in the mouth. The feeling is described as softer, smoother, silkier or slicker. According to Dr Utekhin from Russia, the water becomes structured. What this means is that the bond angles of the two hydrogen atoms hanging onto the oxygen atom change their configuration making the molecule become narrower. This makes it easier for the water molecule to pass through the aqua pores in the cell membrane and thus water is more easily absorbed into the cells. I sense there may be much more going on due to a potential change in pH, which affects the charge on the water molecule.

Here are some of the effects attributed to structured water. It exhibits antibacterial properties, purifies the body and blood by eliminating foreign proteins, and, though the reduction in cholesterol is modest, it still offers some benefits. Additionally, it enhances metabolism. Another aspect in the Russian findings revealed a decrease and fragmentation of gallstones and kidney stones. The crystal structures of these stones, loosely held together, react with water flowing through them, promoting a biochemical reactivity that loosens their bonds, ultimately causing them to dissolve. Moreover, structured water also stimulates the immune system.

In regard to charged water's antibacterial properties, I've found that algae will not grow in the bottles I use. Other bottles I stored water in all eventually grew algae if the water was never charged in them. I also have a friend who commercially grows exotic plants. He says cuttings root two to three times faster in charged water. I've also heard of people charging their fruit with PEMF and been told it makes the fruit taste better and also last longer.

CHAPTER 2
How PEMF Therapy Works

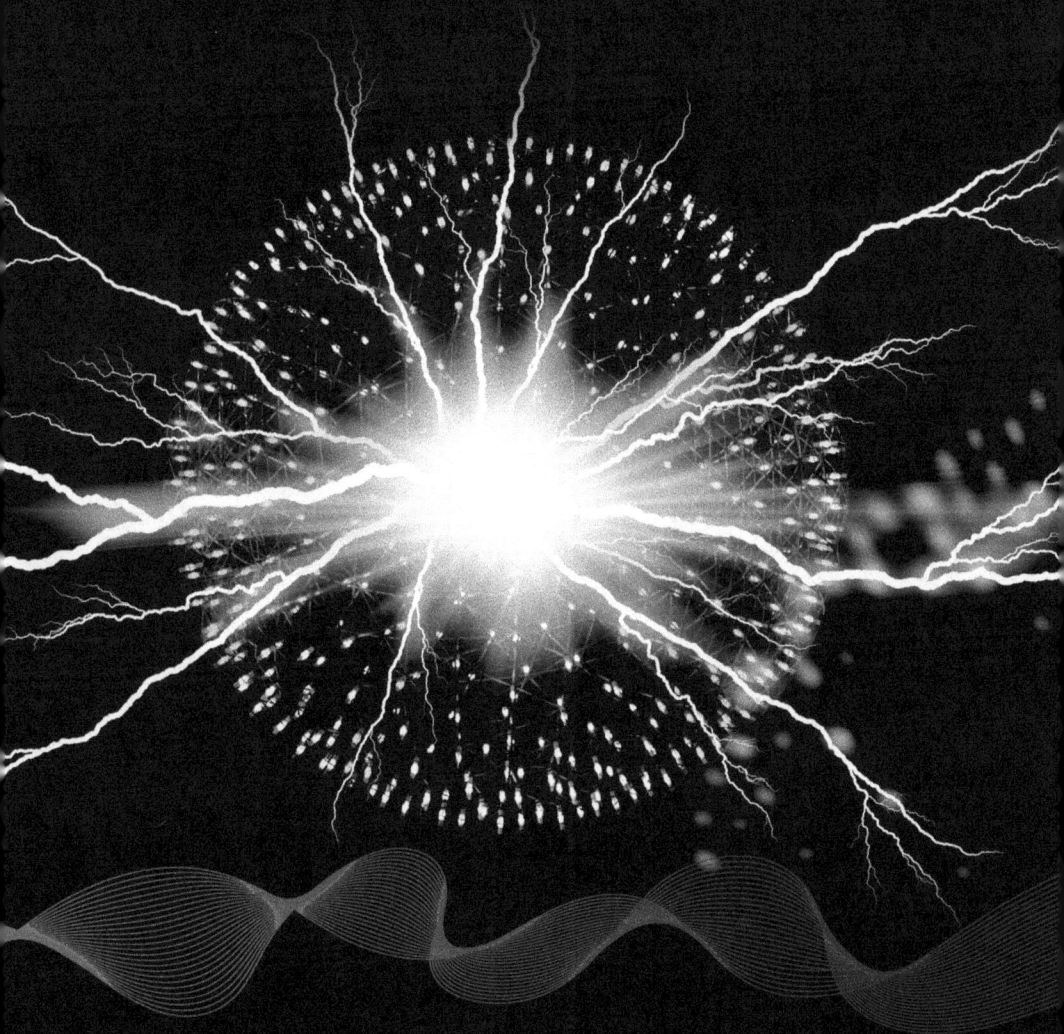

CHAPTER 2
How PEMF Therapy Works

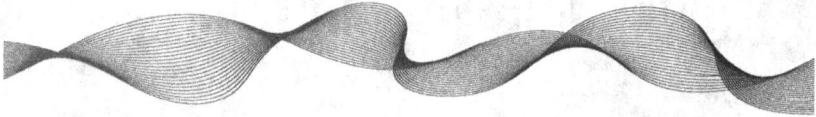

PEMF therapy is still regarded as an innovative approach to health rejuvenation and maintenance. In fact, it's not that innovative at all. PEMF has been commercially available in Europe for nearly thirty years. It has gained recognition and popularity as a non-invasive and effective therapy during the recent decade. This is due to the internet and the increasing interest in frequency technologies by health professionals and the general public. There are thousands of peer-reviewed, double-blind, placebo-controlled studies on PEMF showing benefits for over one hundred health conditions.

The most common question I hear over and over again from people who have experienced the benefits of PEMF is: 'Why doesn't everyone know about this?' It's a good question and one of the reasons for this book.

PEMF in a Nutshell

Here's how PEMF works at a general level and why it all makes sense.

1 - Many chronic illnesses and injuries have an associated low cellular voltage as one contributing factor of the condition. There may also be other contributing factors. Health is about balance and having too much of *anything* or not enough of your core requirements can lead to physiological imbalances. PEMF addresses cellular voltage deficiency or a lack of electrons (energy). PEMF is like an electron multivitamin for energy and increased cellular efficiency, which is why it benefits so many different conditions. There are thousands of clinical studies showing that PEMF improves many different kinds of disorders or imbalances.

2 - As we age, our cellular voltage decreases. In 2011 a study showed that on average, a 65 to 80-year-old has approximately 48% of the voltage of an 18 to 25-year-old. This is exactly why older people don't usually have as much energy as younger people. It's simply because they have less cellular voltage. It's very comparable to the charge in a battery. It you have half the charge then you aren't going to get nearly as far or go as fast during the day as someone else who is younger. It's also why it takes longer for things to heal. It's that very charge or voltage that governs how fast we heal as you will read later in this chapter.

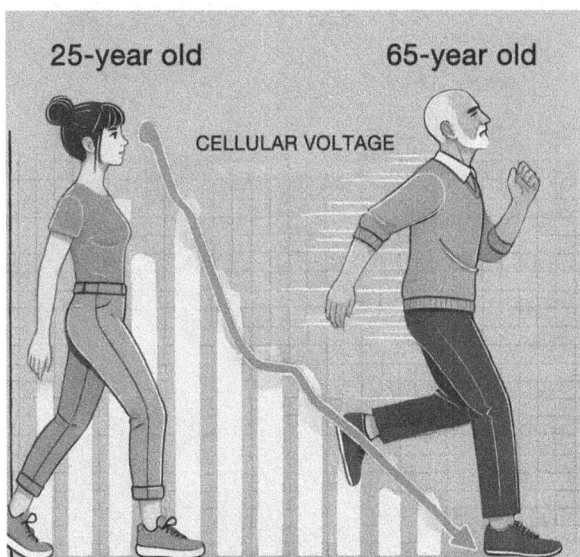

Both of the examples above (chronic conditions/injuries or aging) are associated with bioelectrical blockages or deficiencies of cellular voltage.

There may be other contributing factors such as:

- Nutritional deficiencies
- Pharmaceuticals (side effects)
- Stress
- Diet
- Parasites
- Toxins and other environmental factors like EMFs
- Mental and emotional imbalance
- Genetics

3 - Cellular voltage supplies the energy (electrons) to the bioelectrical network, which is like the operating system software of a computer. Cellular voltage and the bioelectrical network play a crucial role in governing and regulating much of the physiological processes to various degrees in the body such as:

- Overall bioelectrical communication
- Cell growth
- Cell differentiation (cells developing into other specific types of cells
- Apoptosis (programmed cell death)
- Organ development
- Tissue regeneration
- Wound healing
- Immune response
- pH balance
- Circulation

4 - Your cells are like a battery. They have a measurable charge. A low cellular charge or a low voltage, just like a low battery, is not going to be as efficient in running your body's bioelectrical network or you main operating system.

5 - PEMF is a cellular charging system. PEMF uses the same physics as a generator to increase the electrical charge and therefore the bioelectrical efficiency of the body. It works on the same principles as an external pad charger for your phone. The natural, earth-based low frequency waves penetrate every cell in the body and induce microcurrents to charge every cell all at the same time. This is why PEMF works for so many different health issues because:

- Any chronic illness or injury has a low voltage
- As we age our cellular voltage decrease
- Cellular voltage governs many primary functions of the body

Frequency, Intensity & Waveforms

I'll try to keep this simple, but it's good to know some of the fundamental basics of PEMF.

Electromagnetic waves travel very similar to sound or waves on the water. Water is a slow medium; sound is faster and electromagnetic waves travel at the speed of light. You will hear the words frequency, intensity and waveform spoken in the world of PEMF, so it's good to have some understanding of the terms. You don't have to be a physicist, but you still need to be comfortable with the concepts.

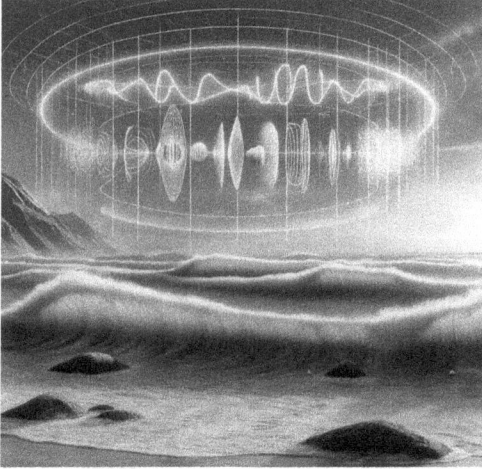

Let's use the ocean waves as an example to get more familiar with the terms. The *frequency* of the waves would be how often each incoming wave crest breaks on the beach. If the waves break every 10 seconds, then the frequency would be 6 times per minute. Hertz (Hz) is the symbol, which is a measure of the number of times *per second*. 6 Hz equals a frequency of a six times per second. Obviously, ocean waves are a much lower frequency.

Intensity would be the height of the wave. Intensity correlates with how much energy is carried in the wave. With water, it's the height of the wave and a ten-meter wave has far more moving weight and therefore more energy in it than a half-meter wave. If it was a sound wave, it would be the volume.

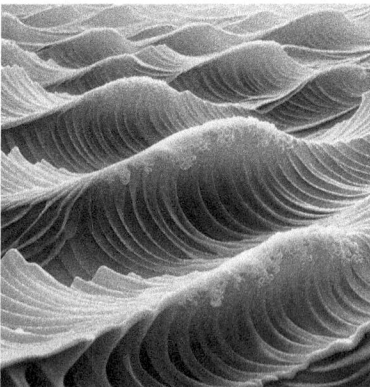

Waveform simply has to do with the shape of the wave. With water, it's very common to see what we call a sine wave with gently sloping peaks and troughs as you normally see in the ocean when looking out away from the shore.

So that's it. You can use the ocean as your metaphor for frequency (number of waves hitting the beach per unit of time), intensity (height of the wave) and waveform (shape of the wave).

Schumann Resonance & Coherence

A common inclination for people first getting interested in PEMF is to become fixated on a specific frequency or intensity range. They believe it to be a magical, sacred or research-proven frequency solution for a particular health issue. In my opinion, there is no one-size-fits-all solution for frequency and intensity in healing the body using PEMF. There's definitely a window or relatively defined range of frequencies and intensities that the cells respond favorably to PEMF. It's just that I've found that everyone responds a bit differently.

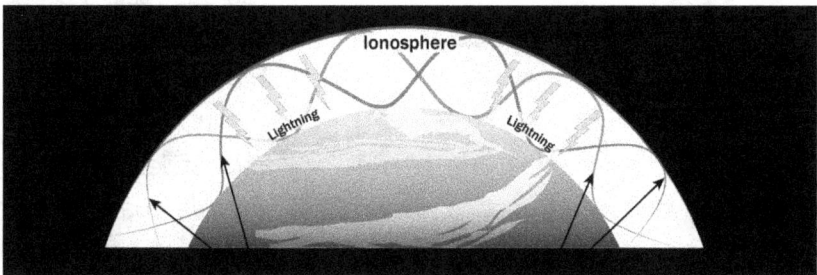

A very common focus of interest is the Schumann resonance. The Schumann resonance is the natural electromagnetic field surrounding the Earth. It is a set of spectrum peaks between 3 Hz and 60 Hz in the extremely low-frequency (ELF) portion of the Earth's electromagnetic field. It's important to note it is not one specific frequency commonly stated as 8.73 Hz.

The primary source of the Schumann Resonance is lightning. It's created by the seven to eight million lightning strikes that happen every day around the world. When lightning occurs, it produces electromagnetic waves that propagate through the Earth's ionosphere cavity, creating a range of frequencies. The Earth's surface and the conductive ionosphere act as boundaries for this cavity, creating a natural electromagnetic resonator. The fundamental Schumann Resonance frequency peak is approximately 7.83 Hz with higher harmonic multiples of the fundamental frequency peaks, such as 14.3 Hz, 20.8 Hz, 27.3 and 33.8 Hz and so on. It is sometimes referred to as the Earth's heartbeat.

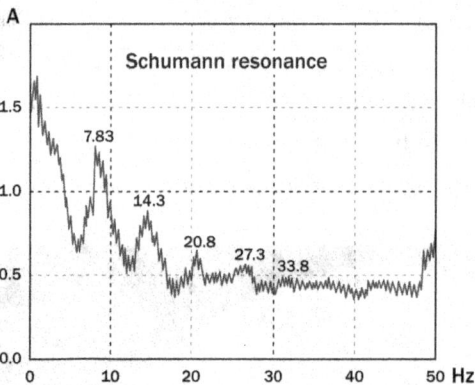

The 7.83 Hz peak has the strongest intensity with the higher harmonic frequencies diminishing in strength. There is really no one magic or specific frequency but a spectrum of frequencies within the biological window of resonance. These are safe, natural, low frequency and low intensity electromagnetic waves. The wave frequencies fall mainly within .1 and 50Hz, but they can go above it up to 100 Hz and a bit beyond. The brain generates frequencies between .01 Hz and 80 Hz. The heart generates frequencies between .05 to 100 Hz.

It's interesting that the electromagnetic emission from healer's hands can now be measured with an ultra-sensitive superconducting quantum interference device called a SQUID magnetometer. Several researchers in the 90's investigated the strong pulsating bio-magnetic field that emanates from the hands of energy practitioners while they work on people. They found the electromagnetic field can be as much as one thousand times greater than the electromagnetic field that normally radiates out from the body. This biofield radiates out an average distance of 1.5 meters.

Additionally, the SQUID magnetometer measured the frequencies coming out of the hands of energy medicine practitioners. It was found to be in the low frequencies ranging from 0.3 Hz to 30 Hz. The frequency signals emitted from their hands were not steady but moved through a 0.3 Hz to 30 Hz range with an average of around 7-8 Hz, which interestingly centers close to the first peak of the Schumann resonance.

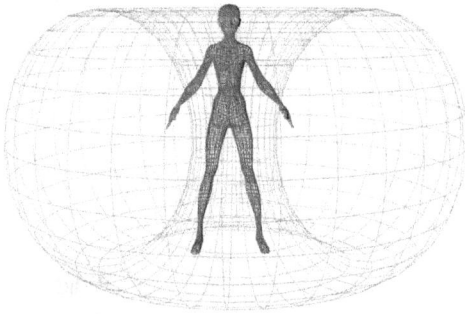

In addition, they found that the brain wave patterns of the practitioner and the patient become synchronized in the alpha state frequencies. This is an excellent example of resonance, which can also create coherence in the whole body. They also found that they pulse in unison with the earth's magnetic field or the Schuman Resonance. Independent medical research has shown that this range of frequencies stimulates healing in the body. In fact, certain frequencies were found to be more suitable for different tissues. For example, 2 Hz encourages nerve regeneration, 7 Hz stimulates bone growth, 10Hz ligament mending and 15 Hz capillary formation.

Resonant Frequencies of Tissues

Frequency	Effect	Reference
1Hz	Melatonin secretion	Lerchl et al., 1998
2Hz	Nerve regeneration	Sisken & Walker, 1995
5Hz	Osteogenesis	Matsunaga et al., 1996
6.4Hz	Cartilage	Sakai et al., 1991
7Hz	Bone growth	Sisken & Walker, 1995
10Hz	Ligament healing	Sisken & Walker, 1995
10Hz	Cell growth	Miyagi et al., 2000
10Hz	Osteogenesis	Matsunaga et al., 1996
10Hz	Collagen production	Lin et al., 1993
10Hz	DNA synthesis	Takahashi et al., 1996
15Hz	Fibroblast proliferation	Sisken & Walker, 1995
15Hz	Osteoporosis	Takayama et al., 1990
20Hz	Osteogenesis	Matsunaga et al., 1996
25Hz	Synergistic effect with nerve growth factor	Sisken & Walker, 1995
40/116Hz	Inflammation	Reilly et al., n.d.
50Hz	Osteogenesis	Matsunaga et al., 1996

One of the reasons I like the triple sawtooth waveform, which the whole body mat generates on my system, is because it delivers a rich and harmonic spectrum of low frequencies and intensities within the biological window of resonance. These frequencies match or resonant with all the different frequencies and intensities of the cells in the body. Waveforms, like the triple sawtooth, will be discussed later in the book.

It's very understandable that people are very attracted to the Schumann resonance or the 'heartbeat of the earth.' There's no getting around the fact that it's the predominate frequency of healer's hands. Also remember, there is more than one Schumann frequency. As an aside, it would be very interesting to measure the frequency of a surgeon's hand along with the hands of a mother holding a baby.

There is a synchronicity with the earth's natural heartbeat frequency and the frequency of a healer's hands. But, it's only one of many different frequencies that resonant with the body. Plus, as I've said, everyone is different, because what frequency resonates with one person can be different with what resonates with another person. In this case I'm talking about the whole person and not specific body tissues. The Schumann frequencies are definitely a good place to start. By that, I mean using a full spectrum of low frequencies in and around the full range of all of the peaks of the Schuman resonance to treat the whole body. PEMF devices where you set one specific frequency fail on the resonance score board as they will not address the full biological window of resonance of the cells. You would have to run through each program a minimum of at least thirty times for each individual frequency to get a full spectrum of 0 to 30 Hz. Fortunately, the system I use broadcasts a full spectrum of frequencies in the biological range.

Every once in a while, I get the opportunity to treat what I call a really sensitive person. What I mean is someone having a refined and keen awareness of energy, vibrations… call it what you may. Many times, they are energy workers or healers. Reiki people are very sensitive along with kinesiologists to name just a few. They can actually feel the very low intensity PEMF pulses. Generally, most people don't feel anything with low intensity systems, but, around 10% of people do feel the subtle pulses of the electromagnetic waves. Around 25% can sometimes feel a slight tingling, usually in a problem area, but they can't feel the actual pulsing. With low intensity systems, there are no dramatic muscles contractions that occur with high intensity systems.

Taking it up to another level, some of these 'sensitives' have the ability to measure or feel the resonance happening within the cells in their body. It happens predominantly with the intensity setting and not so much with variations in frequency. Intensity controls how much charge is generated in the cells. Across the board, almost every one of these people I've spoken to *all* prefer the three lowest intensities the PEMF system can produce. This is where they 'feel' the resonance occurring within them. Less is more, as you will learn later in the book.

"Modern biophysics research has confirmed that tissues respond to very tiny energy fields of the appropriate frequency, intensity and pulse shape. If you are not getting results, try less energy or shorter treatments."

– James L Oschman author of 'Energy Medicine.'

With intensity, most people have a tendency to think that more is better. There is a way another that I've found to be enlightened by the importance of low intensities in regard to creating resonance within the cells.

Resonance refers to the phenomenon where cells and biological systems exhibit a strong and positive response to electromagnetic energy. Another way one can think of resonance is being in tune or being in the same key if we were talking about sound waves (music) instead of electromagnetic waves.

As an example, when two identical tuning forks are near each other, resonance may be demonstrated. If one of the tuning forks is struck and begins to vibrate, it produces sound waves at its key frequency. When the sound waves reach the second tuning fork, they exert a force at the same frequency at which the fork naturally vibrates. If the frequency of the incoming sound waves matches the natural frequency of the second tuning fork, it starts to vibrate in sympathy. The vibrations of the second tuning fork reinforce and synchronize with the vibrations of the first tuning fork.

As a result of this resonance, the sound produced by the two vibrating tuning forks becomes louder and more distinct. The energy transfer between the two tuning forks allows for the amplification and enhancement of the vibrations and sound.

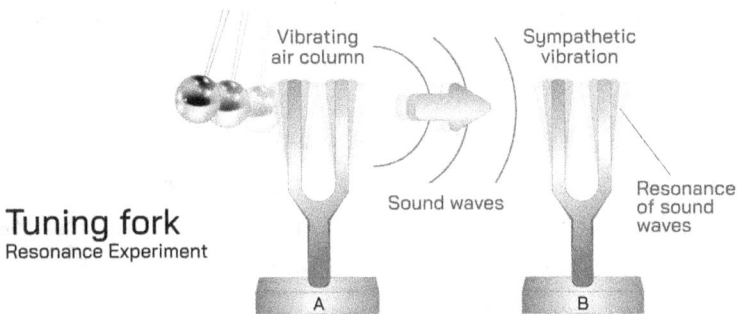

Vibrating air column

Sympathetic vibration

Sound waves

Resonance of sound waves

Tuning fork
Resonance Experiment

A

B

Just like the two tuning forks, the cells in your body respond positively to electromagnetic frequencies that are capable of producing a resonance. Every cell vibrates at a different frequency or has a different window of resonance where it will respond positively. This can vary from one person to the next to a degree. The cells within an organ will also have different frequencies depending on their form, functionality and their present energetic state. Therefore, to cover all bases, it's best to generate a spectrum or range of low frequencies that covers the biological window of response or what's also known as the "Adey window." Dr. James Oschman refers to it as the 'power/frequency window,' the relatively narrow range of signal properties that will produce a maximum resonating biological effect.

Dr. Ross Adey (Adey window) was a prominent pioneering researcher in bio-electromagnetics during the 1960s and the 1970s. He discovered a narrow range of electromagnetic frequencies, typically around *0.1 to 30 Hertz*, at which cells and tissues exhibit heightened sensitivity and response to external electromagnetic signals. This sensitivity is due to resonance effects and the ability of these frequencies to influence cellular processes including improved ion transport and cell signaling. These findings led to investigations into the potential therapeutic applications in various medical contexts, such as promoting tissue repair, bone healing and the treatment for certain neurological conditions.

People search the internet and find research studies on a particular disorder. If a certain study used a particular frequency, waveform or intensity, then they automatically jump to the conclusion that this is what they need because the study achieved some kind of favorable result. It's only for research purposes that fixed frequencies must be selected in order to define the specific parameters of the system's outputs as precisely as possible. It doesn't mean all the chosen parameters are the ultimate solution for everyone in regard to frequency, intensity or the waveform. Those parameters were simply what was chosen for the study, but it may be a really good place to start.

As previously stated, resonance occurs when the frequency of an external stimulus matches the natural frequency or resonant frequency of a cell, tissue or an organ system. When an external stimulus such as electromagnetic waves harmonize with the same resonant frequency

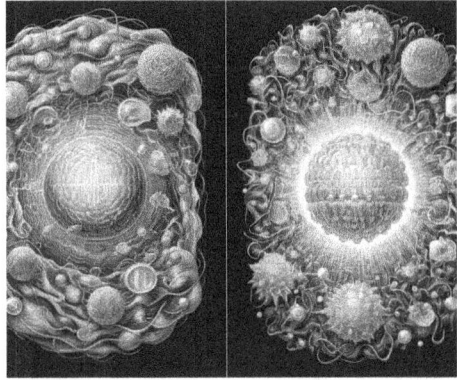

Incoherence vs. Coherence

of a cellular component, it can induce a more pronounced and favorable response, enhancing cellular processes and improving cellular communication. This in turn can create coherence.

Coherence, in the context of cellular resonance, refers to the synchronization or alignment of cellular activities and processes, particularly on the level of electromagnetic frequencies. When cellular components (organs in the body) or whole systems are in a state of coherence, their frequencies and oscillations become harmonized by being in phase. This means that the timing of the peaks and troughs of the waves are aligned, leading to a more efficient and integrated functioning of the whole cellular network. It's analogous to a symphony orchestra all playing together and precisely synchronized in time and in the same key.

In a coherent state, cells within a tissue or organism are better able to communicate and synchronize their activities with each other. This coherence can be achieved through various mechanisms, including the alignment of cellular frequencies and the establishment of coherent electromagnetic fields within and around cells. Low frequency and low intensity PEMF therapy induces resonance and the corresponding coherence by delivering harmonious and natural electromagnetic fields to all the cells in the body.

pH and Voltage

The connection between pH (the acidity or alkalinity of your body) and cellular voltage is paramount to understanding and explaining one of the fundamental reasons PEMF therapy works so well for so many different imbalances within the body.

To better understand the connection between pH and voltage, it's best to define what each term means:

1. **pH:** pH stands for 'potential hydrogen,' which is a measure of the concentration of hydrogen ions (H+) present in a substance. In simple terms, pH is a measure of the acidity or alkalinity of a substance. The pH scale ranges from 0 to 14 with 7 being neutral and values below 7 indicating acidity and values above 7 indicating alkalinity.

2. **Voltage**: In 1927 Noble Prize Laureate, Dr. Otto Warburg, discovered that human cells have a measurable voltage just like a battery. Cellular voltage is a measure of the potential difference in the charge levels between the inside and outside of the cell membrane called the transmembrane potential. Cellular voltage is typically measured in millivolts (mV). That's in thousandths of a volt. AA batteries are 1.5 volts or 1,500 millivolts (mV). Your cells' voltage is 20 to 25 millivolts.

Cellular Voltage & pH (acidity/alkalinity)

1.5 volts = 1,500 mV (millivolts)

ALKALINE	Cell Voltage (millivolts)	
A	-50 mV	New Cells Created
L		
K	-40 mV / -30 mV	Children
A		
	-25 mV / -20 mV	Healthy Adults
L		
I	-15 mV	Tired & Low Energy
N	-10 mV	Illness
E	-5 mV	Pain & Inflammation
	0	
Acidic Terrain	5 mv	Pathogenic

Cells, like a battery, have a voltage. With age or illness, the voltage decreases. Therefore cell efficiency declines so the body can't maintain or restore health.

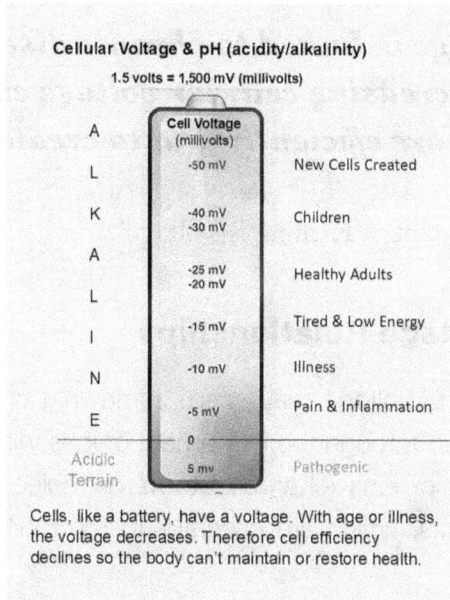

Healthy human cells operate most efficiently in an environment with a pH of 7.35 to 7.45, which corresponds to a voltage of approximately -20 mV (millivolts) to -25 mV. The negative sign (-) indicates a negative charge or the addition of electrons. -25 mV is 25 one thousandth of one volt (25/1000 or .025 volts. Although this voltage is 60 times less than that of an AA battery, its small value does not diminish the importance of its potential for life itself. This *is* the very spark of life, which in my opinion is *the* fundamental energy running the whole show… meaning your life force.

A normal or healthy cellular voltage facilitates the automatic entry of oxygen into cells, which is essential for maintaining optimal health. Conversely, as oxygen levels decline, so does overall well-being. Chronic diseases are often associated with a low cellular voltage potential or a depletion of voltage *and* a low oxygen (anaerobic) environment. Usually, if you have one, then you have the other.

"Low voltage is linked to chronic disease and injuries. Increasing cellular voltage enables the cells run more efficiently and to create healthy new cells."
– Dr. Jerry Tennant – 'Healing is Voltage'

The pH-Voltage Relationship

Although pH and voltage may seem somewhat distinct, they are intrinsically linked through the movement of ions within our bodies. The movement of ions (charged atoms or molecules) generates electrical currents, which are essential to run many physiological processes.

In our bodies, the movement of hydrogen ions (H+) is particularly significant. When hydrogen ions are involved, the transfer of a positive charge occurs, which creates a voltage potential or an increased charge. Therefore, changes in pH levels reflect changes in the electrical potential within our bodies.

In other words, alterations in the concentration of hydrogen ions (pH) directly affect the electrical potential (voltage) in our cells and tissues. This interconnectedness highlights the innate relationship between pH and voltage, emphasizing their fundamental role in maintaining the healthy functioning of our physiological systems. *Simply stated, if you increase the pH of the body, you increase the cellular voltage. On the other hand, if you increase the cellular voltage using PEMF, then you increase the pH.*

An important point to remember about PEMF is that electromagnetic waves penetrate every cell in the body. *Therefore, if you increase cellular voltage using PEMF, then you are increasing the pH and alkalizing every cell in the body all at once.* Furthermore, if you are aware of how important alkalinity is to creating a healthy environment in the body, then you are on the road to seeing why PEMF helps so many different kinds of health issues.

One important consideration is that any cellular charge and increase in pH from a PEMF treatment will last approximately six hours, depending on the hydration of the body. The more hydrated, the longer the cellular charge is held. Again, this is very analogous to charging a battery. Ideally, if you owned a system, you'd charge your body a couple of times per day to keep your pH alkaline, oxygenate your cells and maintain your increased cellular efficiencies.

Cell Voltage in Health & Disease

Average Cell Voltage in Milli-Volts (mV)

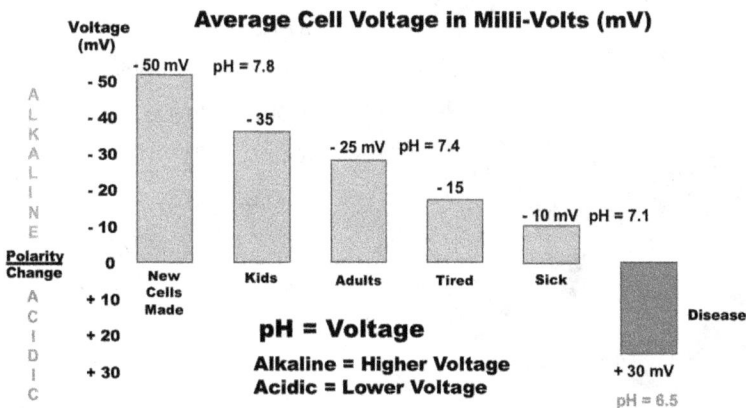

A healthy adult has an approximate pH of 7.4 and therefore a voltage of -25 mV(millivolts). Kids have a higher voltage of around -35 mV, so in effect, *they do have more energy.* To make a healthy new cell takes approximately -50 mV. As you get tired or sick, your voltage decreases. Most major disorders have an even lower voltage, which drops below the pH level of 7 and turns acidic with a + charge. A + charge means there is a lack of electrons. Electrons, which are basically energy, are what you want to have in abundance. Electrons have a negative charge.

Cellular voltage is one of the primary governing factors that controls the physiological efficiency of healing and health maintenance. It makes sense to give yourself a cellular charge a couple of times a day to keep your cellular efficiency up along with your pH. Over time, this will pay some of the best dividends. PEMF is being used more and more by individuals who recognize the benefits of taking proactive control of their own health.

The Spark of Life: Cellular Voltage

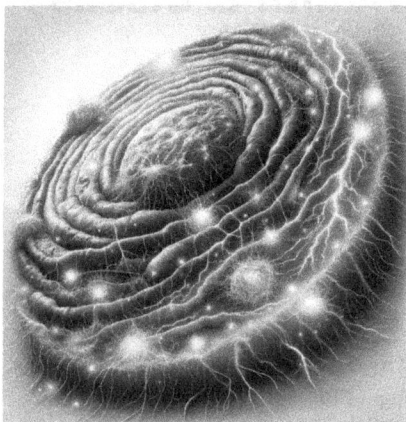

In 2011, Richard Nuccitelli invented the Dermacorder®, which measures the tiny electrical fields surrounding a wound. When a bodily wound or injury occurs, the electric field or voltage immediately peaks around the area of the wound. As the wound heals over time, the voltage surrounding the wound slowing declines to the baseline voltage level of the neighboring healthy tissues. The increased voltage enhances or boosts the biochemical and the bioelectrical healing processes in the wound. It's the increased voltage that is one of the driving or governing forces to speed the healing of the wound.

"There's not a day goes by that I don't do PEMF."

– Tony Robbins, author of Life Force

Your overall bioelectrical potential, or your body's cellular charge, operates as the primary governing force in our bodies. It is one of the major contributing factors that determines the efficiency of repairing, restoring and maintaining health.

This internal battery charge regulates metabolism, biochemistry, communication signaling and is essentially the spark of life as Dr Michael Levin calls it. Levin, the director at Tufts University Center for Regenerative and Developmental Biology, is known for his work in the field of regenerative biology and developmental bioelectricity.

Levin has proposed the concept of a non-neural bioelectrical system. This theory proposes that electrical signals play a crucial role in governing and regulating various biological processes beyond the nervous system. Levin describes the non-neural bioelectrical network as the main software controlling multiple levels of programming throughout the body.

Levin characterizes the genes as the body's architectural hardware. He says that it's the bioelectrical network that serves as the system software of your physiology. My theory is that if the bioelectrical network isn't running at a sufficient level or threshold of efficiency, then the body does not function and communicate effectively. Therefore, it has difficulty maintaining or restoring health.

Here's a general overview of how this system works, its functions and its importance:

1. **Electrical Signaling in Non-Neural Tissues:** While the nervous system primarily relies on electrical signals for communication between neurons, non-neural tissues also exhibit tremendous amounts of bioelectrical activity. This activity involves the movement and communication of electrically charged particles (ions) across cell membranes.

2. **Ion Channels and Membrane Potential:** Cells in non-neural tissues possess channels in their membranes, allowing ions such as sodium, potassium, calcium and chloride to flow in and out of the cell. This movement of ions creates changes in membrane voltage, which can propagate electrical signals within and between cells.

3. **Cellular Communication:** Bioelectrical signals in non-neural tissues serve as a means of communication between cells and tissues. These signals can influence various cellular processes, including cell proliferation, differentiation, migration and apoptosis (programmed cell death).

4. **Regulation of Physiological Processes:** The non-neural bioelectrical system plays a vital role in regulating physiological processes across different organ systems. It helps coordinate organ development, tissue regeneration, wound healing and immune responses. Additionally, bioelectrical signals are involved in the control of ion homeostasis, pH balance and fluid movement within the body.

5. **Emergent Properties and Pattern Formation:** One of the intriguing aspects of the non-neural bioelectrical system is its ability to give rise to emergent properties and complex patterns of biological organization. Electrical signals can orchestrate the formation of anatomical structures during development and

contribute to the maintenance of tissue integrity and function in adulthood. There is an intrinsic intelligence to it all.

6. **Importance in Regenerative Medicine:** Understanding and manipulating the bioelectrical properties of cells and tissues hold significant potential for regenerative medicine and tissue engineering. Researchers are exploring how electrical stimulation, ion channel modulation and bioelectric signaling can be harnessed to promote tissue repair and regeneration in various medical conditions and injuries.

How Voltage Regulates the Body

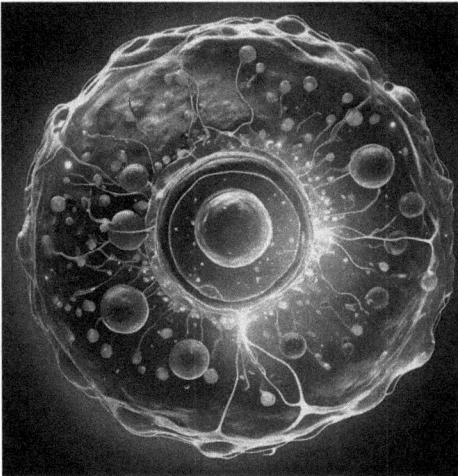

The way bioelectrical charges govern the biochemistry in the body is related to the role of electrical signals in cellular and also in physiological processes. The body is a very complex system of cells. The fundamental unit of communication within and between cells involves the movement of ions, which are electrically 'charged' particles. A lower overall cellular charge, reflected as a reduced cell membrane potential, can decrease the efficiency of the cell in maintaining a healthy internal environment and also decrease cellular communication with the neighboring cells.

"All energy is electromagnetic in nature. Nothing happens in the body without an electromagnetic exchange. Electromagnetic energy controls the chemistry in the body. Disruption of electromagnetic energy in cells causes impaired cell metabolism."

– Dr. William Pawluk

Cellular processes and functions that rely on proper ion movement and membrane potential (cellular charge) may be compromised, potentially leading to cellular dysfunction. In severe cases, it may result in cell damage or death. Maintaining an appropriate membrane potential or cellular charge is vital for the overall health and functionality of cells in various tissues and organs throughout the body.

1. **Cell Membrane Potential:**

   - The outer membrane of cells, known as the cell membrane, plays a crucial role in maintaining a bioelectrical charge. The cell membrane is selectively permeable, meaning it allows specific ions to pass through while restricting others.

   - The movement of ions across the cell membrane generates a voltage difference, which is known as the membrane potential. This membrane potential is essential for various cellular functions.

2. **Action Potentials:**

   - Nerve cells (neurons) are particularly important in this context. They use electrical signals called action potentials to transmit information over long distances.

- An action potential is a rapid change in membrane potential that travels along the neuron. It is initiated by the movement of ions, such as sodium and potassium, across the cell membrane.

3. Ion Channels:

- Ion channels are proteins embedded in the cell membrane that allow the selective passage of specific ions. The opening and closing of these ion channels are often controlled by changes in the voltage across the membrane.

- Ion channels play a crucial role in transmitting signals within neurons, as well as in the communication between neurons and other cells, such as muscle cells.

4. Neurotransmitter Release:

- At synapses, which are the junctions between neurons, the electrical signal is converted into a chemical signal. When an action potential reaches the end of a neuron, it triggers the release of neurotransmitters into the synaptic cleft.

- The neurotransmitters then bind to receptors on the adjacent cell, leading to changes in its membrane potential and initiating a new electrical signal.

5. Muscle Contraction:

- In muscle cells, the bioelectrical charge is crucial for initiating muscle contractions. The release of calcium ions within muscle cells, triggered by electrical signals, is a key step in the contraction process.

6. Cellular Metabolism:

- The bioelectrical environment also influences cellular metabolism. For example, certain ions are involved in the regulation of enzyme activity, which, in turn, affects biochemical reactions within cells.

7. Cellular Communication:

- The bioelectrical charge, specifically the membrane potential in neurons, is vital for transmitting signals throughout the nervous system. Neurons rely on changes in membrane potential to generate action potentials, which allow for the rapid and precise transmission of information.

8. Metabolism and Enzyme Activity:

- The bioelectrical environment of cells influences the activity of enzymes, which are essential for biochemical reactions. Enzymes often function optimally within a specific range of ion concentrations and membrane potentials. Deviations from these optimal conditions can affect metabolic processes.

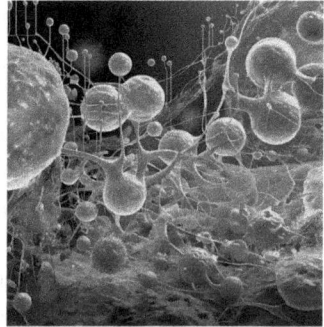

9. Cellular Transport:

- Ion channels, which are integral to the bioelectrical charge, play a crucial role in the transport of ions and molecules across cell membranes. Proper ion transport is essential for maintaining cell volume, osmotic balance, and the overall stability of cellular environments.

10. Cell Signaling:

- Cellular communication and signaling pathways often involve changes in the bioelectrical charge. For example, the opening and closing of ion channels are central to the reception and transmission of signals that regulate cell growth, differentiation and responses to external stimuli.

In conclusion, the bioelectrical charge of cells, particularly the membrane potential, is directly connected with the biochemistry of the body. It governs processes such as signal transmission in neurons, muscle contraction and cellular metabolism. The intricate interplay between bioelectricity and biochemistry is fundamental to the functioning of living organisms.

Effects of Low Cellular Voltage:

1. Impaired Nerve Function:

- A low bioelectrical charge can lead to impaired nerve function, affecting the transmission of signals between neurons. This can result in issues such as numbness, tingling or muscle weakness.

2. Muscle Weakness and Fatigue:

- Inadequate bioelectrical charge can compromise the ability of muscles to contract efficiently, leading to weakness and fatigue.

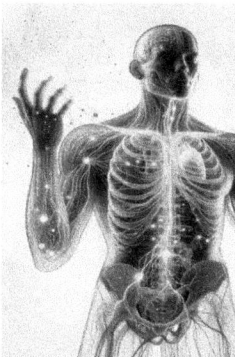

3. Metabolic Dysfunction:

- Changes in the bioelectrical environment can disrupt cellular metabolism, potentially impacting energy production and nutrient processing.

4. Cellular Stress:

- Cells may experience stress and dysfunction when the bioelectrical environment deviates from the optimal range. This can contribute to cellular damage and may be associated with various health conditions.

5. Altered Cellular Signaling:

- Low bioelectrical charge can disrupt cellular signaling pathways, affecting processes such as cell growth, differentiation and response to environmental cues.

6. Poor Sleep, Mental Brain Fog, Irritability

- A low bioelectrical charge during sleep can lead to brain fog and irritability, disrupting cognitive function and mood regulation.

In summary, maintaining an appropriate bioelectrical charge is vital for the proper functioning of cells and the entire body. Deviations from the normal bioelectrical environment can lead to a range of physiological issues, impacting nerve function, muscle contraction, metabolism and overall cellular health.

Bioelectrical System Functions in the Body:

1. The bioelectrical system conducts electrical signals throughout the body.
2. It helps control various physiological processes through electrical impulses.
3. The system coordinates the activities of different organs and tissues.
4. It facilitates muscle contraction through electrical signals.

5. Bioelectrical signals help regulate blood circulation and flow.

6. It sends commands to various parts of the body, directing their actions.

7. The bioelectrical system processes information and computes responses.

8. It converts electrical signals into chemical signals at synapses.

9. The system calibrates the intensity and timing of electrical impulses.

10. It counteracts disruptions in electrical activity to maintain homeostasis.

11. The bioelectrical system helps regulate various physiological processes.

12. It integrates signals from different parts of the body.

13. The system modulates the intensity and frequency of electrical impulses.

14. It maintains the balance of ions and electrical gradients within cells.

15. Bioelectric signals serve as communication between cells and tissues.

16. It transmits information across neural and non-neural pathways.

17. Bioelectricity influences cellular behavior and tissue organization.

18. The system adapts to changing environmental conditions and stimuli.

19. It enables cells and tissues to respond to internal and external cues.

20. Bioelectric signals synchronize the activities of different cell populations.

Voltage Storage in the Body

Where It's Stored:

Cellular voltage, often referred to as membrane potential, is primarily stored across the cell membranes. This voltage is crucial for various cellular functions and is maintained by the distribution of ions, such as sodium (Na+), potassium (K+), calcium (Ca2+), and chloride (Cl-), across the cell membrane.

The main areas where voltage is stored and utilized include:

1. **Cell Membranes:** The lipid bilayer of the cell membrane creates a separation of charges, leading to a voltage difference across the membrane.

2. **Mitochondria:** These organelles have their own membrane potential, essential for ATP production through a unique oxidative cellular energy production process.

3. **Piezoelectric Effect in Muscle Contraction:** The piezoelectric effect refers to the ability of certain materials to generate an electric charge in response to applied mechanical stress. In the context of human physiology, this phenomenon plays a crucial role in muscle function and energy generation.

Muscles act as the major storage facility for cellular voltage. They also generate voltage through piezoelectricity, which occurs when muscles are stretched or compressed during movement, which creates an electrical charge.

How the Piezoelectric Effect Works in Muscles:

1. Muscle Composition:

- Muscles are composed of piezoelectric materials, such as collagen and elastin. These materials have the ability to generate electric charges when they are compressed, stretched, or otherwise mechanically stressed.

2. Mechanism During Muscle Contraction:

- When muscles contract, they undergo mechanical deformation. This deformation creates a mechanical stress on the piezoelectric materials within the muscle fibers.

- As the muscle fibers are compressed and stretched during contraction and relaxation, they generate small electrical charges.

3. Generation of Electrical Energy:

- The electrical charges generated by the piezoelectric effect contribute to the overall bioelectric field of the body. This field plays a crucial role in various physiological processes, including cellular communication, repair and regeneration.

4. Contribution to Cellular Voltage:

- The electrical energy generated by muscle contractions helps maintain and enhance the voltage across cell membranes (membrane potential). This is vital for various cellular functions, including nutrient transport, waste removal, and signal transduction.

- Enhanced membrane potential improves the efficiency of cellular processes and overall cellular health, contributing to better energy management in the body.

Benefits of the Piezoelectric Effect in Muscles:

1. Improved Circulation:

- The electrical charges generated help enhance blood flow and oxygen delivery to tissues, improving overall circulation and nutrient delivery.

2. Enhanced Cellular Function:

- By contributing to the membrane potential, the piezoelectric effect supports efficient cellular function, promoting better energy production and utilization.

3. Tissue Repair and Regeneration:

- The bioelectric fields generated can aid in tissue repair and regeneration, helping the body recover from injuries more effectively.

4. Energy Boost:

- The generation of electrical charges during muscle activity contributes to the body's overall energy levels, providing a natural boost and enhancing physical performance.

Practical Implications:

- Exercise: Regular physical activity and muscle movement are essential for harnessing the benefits of the piezoelectric effect. Activities like walking, running and strength training stimulate muscle contractions and the subsequent generation of electrical charges.

54
www.PEMFINC.com | www.PEMF.com.au

- Therapies: Specific therapies, such as pulsed electromagnetic field (PEMF) therapy, can enhance the natural piezoelectric effect in muscles. PEMF further supports the storage of cellular voltage that can contribute to overall health.

Understanding the piezoelectric effect in muscles underscores the importance of physical activity and movement in maintaining optimal health and energy levels. By leveraging this natural phenomenon, individuals can enhance their body's bioelectric fields, contributing to better overall well-being.

How It's Stored:

The storage of cellular voltage is maintained by:

1. **Ion Pumps:** Such as the sodium-potassium pump ($Na+/K+$ ATPase) which actively transports $Na+$ out of the cell and $K+$ into the cell, using ATP.

2. **Ion Channels:** These channels allow for selective ion flow across the membrane, contributing to the resting membrane potential and action potentials in excitable cells.

3. **Electrochemical Gradients:** The difference in ion concentration inside and outside the cell creates an electrochemical gradient that stores potential energy.

4. **Piezoelectric Effect in Muscles:** The mechanical stress on muscles during movement generates electrical charges, contributing to the body's overall voltage storage.

Increasing or Preventing Loss of Cellular Voltage:

Methods to Increase or Maintain Cellular Voltage:

1. **Nutrition**: Adequate intake of electrolytes such as potassium, sodium, magnesium and calcium are crucial for maintaining ion balance and membrane potential.

2. **Hydration**: Proper hydration ensures optimal ion transport and cellular function. The more hydrated you are, the more cellular voltage you can store.

3. **Antioxidants**: Reducing oxidative stress with antioxidants (vitamins C and E, hydrogen inhalation) can protect cellular structures and maintain membrane integrity.

4. **Exercise**: Regular physical activity enhances mitochondrial function, generates piezoelectric charges in muscles and improves overall cellular health.

5. **Grounding**: Direct contact with the Earth's surface can help restore cellular voltage

6. **PEMF Therapy**: PEMF therapy has been shown to enhance cellular repair processes and improve membrane potential by stimulating ion flow, increasing ATP production and generating microcurrents in the cells.

Preventing Loss of Cellular Voltage:

1. **Avoiding Toxins**: Reducing exposure to environmental toxins, heavy metals and pollutants can prevent cellular damage and loss of membrane potential.

2. **Reducing Inflammation**: Managing chronic inflammation through diet, lifestyle changes and nutritional supplementation can help preserve cellular function.

3. **Stress Management**: Chronic stress can lead to cellular dysfunction. Practices such as meditation, deep breathing and adequate sleep can help maintain cellular health.

4. **Proper Medication Use**: Some medications can affect ion balance and membrane potential. Use medications as prescribed and discuss any concerns with a healthcare provider.

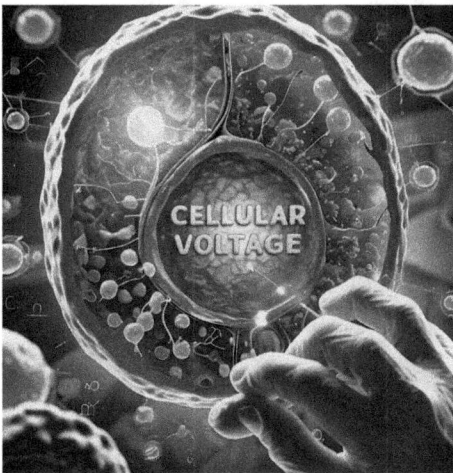

By concentrating on as many of these strategies, we can improve the body's capacity to sustain healthy cellular voltage. This promotes optimal cellular functioning. In closing, one of the easiest and most effective strategies listed above is to drink more water. It's estimated that 80% of people are consistently dehydrated to one degree or another. Dehydration is associated with many different kinds of pathologies, so adding two, three or more glasses per day can make a difference.

CHAPTER 3

The Benefits of PEMF

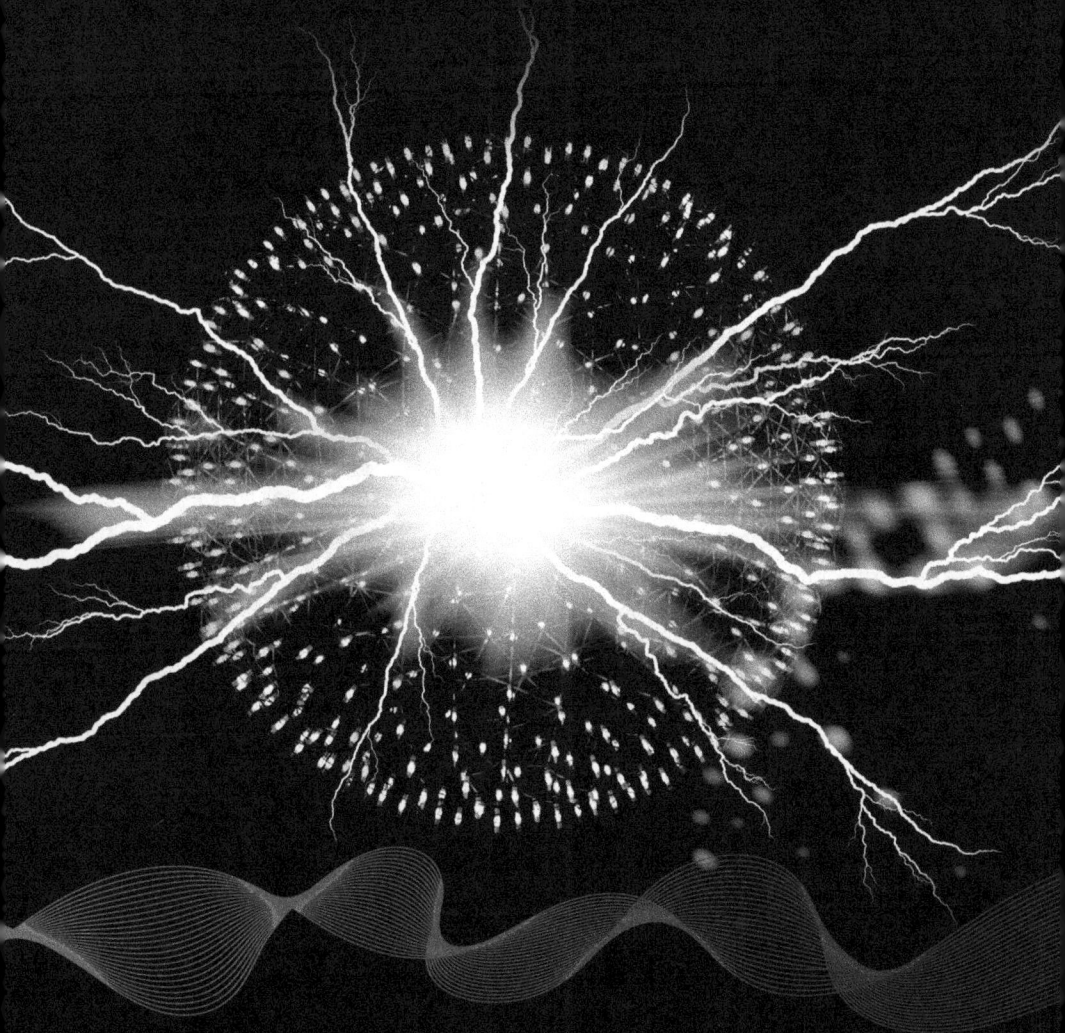

CHAPTER 3
The Benefits of PEMF

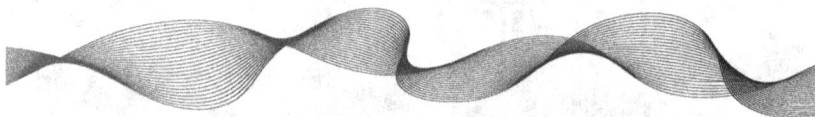

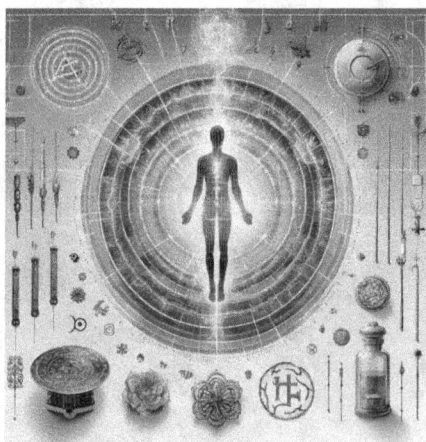

There are many kinds of benefits that come with adopting PEMF therapy into your life. As one looks over the technology available in the current market, I've yet to see *anything* that comes close to achieving the benefits that PEMF therapy provides to people with so many different health conditions. I say this not only looking at the benefits of PEMF but to the ease of use. PEMF can be done in your own home, it's drug-free, non-invasive and safe if low intensities are used. There's also the simplicity of treatment protocols, the thoroughness of reaching every cell in the body and its availability to almost everyone in the world. Still, very few people, relatively speaking, have ever heard of PEMF therapy.

PEMF therapy is simply a cellular recharging system. It addresses a potential bioelectrical deficiency in the body, which is low cellular voltage. Your cells are like a battery with a certain voltage that needs to be maintained. If you get sick, have a chronic condition or are injured, then you most likely have a low cellular voltage in some area of your body as one contributing factor. Yes, you may have other deficiencies, toxins or imbalances of various kinds along with the low cellular voltage. This low voltage can drain the whole body, because everything is connected bio-electrically. Another important contributing factor is that as you age, your cellular voltage decreases. This has been measured. It is one of the fundamental reasons that things take longer to heal in older people.

Cellular voltage is one of the keys, if not THE key driving factor that determines the efficiency and effectiveness of your metabolism, your biochemistry, your immune system and the overall state of your health. For me, PEMF therapy addresses one of the primary deficiencies most people aren't aware that they can supplement: a lack of cellular energy. The word 'energy' is used in many different ways, but in regard to your health, this energy is really cellular voltage, something that is measurable and very real. I like to think of this energy simply as electrons. So PEMF therapy could be thought of as an electron supplementation or an electron (energy) delivery system.

Looking across the landscape in regard to PEMF, I need to say that PEMF isn't perfect and it doesn't work for everyone. Generally speaking, the 80/20 rule comes into play from what I've seen in my experience with treating people. Eighty percent of people will see some level of improvement and twenty percent won't notice anything. Within the twenty percent who don't see any benefits, I've treated others that have realized an improvement for the same health condition. There are too many lifestyle and individual personal variables at play to be able to determine any negative or even positive contributing factors at play. Also, many health practitioners know that a certain percentage of people don't want to get better whether they are consciously aware of it or not.

PEMF Research

Graph of Research Studies on PEMF

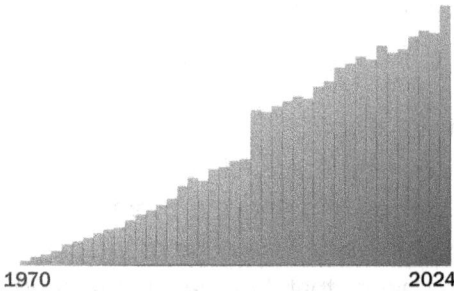

1970   2024

One of the things that first attracted me to PEMF was all the research that backs up the effectiveness of PEMF.

When I first started practicing PEMF, there were twelve or thirteen hundred research studies listed on PubMed. Today there are currently over four thousand studies listed. In total, there have been three to five times as many studies globally. Not all the studies are positive and not all studies find significant benefits, but the majority do find positive results or results that indicate more research or a larger scale needs to take place. PEMF research is becoming more and more popular for research studies.

The Mayo Clinic has been actively involved in exploring the potential clinical uses of PEMF therapy, particularly focusing on its benefits for vascular health and its applications for conditions like pre-diabetes and metabolic syndrome. Their research has highlighted PEMF therapy's ability to improve cellular communication and enhance overall cellular health, contributing to the growing body of evidence supporting the therapeutic benefits of PEMF.

The benefits of pulsed electromagnetic field (PEMF) therapy have been demonstrated through thousands of double-blind, peer-reviewed, placebo-controlled clinical studies done in many countries with many different PEMF devices. As a general rule, the PEMF systems used in the studies are built by the research laboratories. Therefore, commercial systems currently for sale on the market are not used. There are a few studies done by manufacturers, but there is an obvious built-in conflict of interest in the studies paid for by any PEMF manufacturer.

Medical PEMF therapy has been accepted in many countries around the world. The US Food and Drug Administration (FDA) has approved the use of specific PEMF devices in the healing of non-union bone fractures in 1979, urinary incontinence and muscle stimulation in 1998, depression and anxiety unresponsive to pharmaceuticals in 2006 and one form of brain cancer in 2011. Israel has accepted the use of PEMF devices for the treatment of migraine headaches. The European Union has many acceptances for the use of PEMF therapy in many areas including healing and recovery from trauma, degeneration and the treatment of pain associated with these conditions.

The PEMF Benefits List

Reduced Pain

In the US, more than twenty percent of people are living with some kind of chronic pain... the most common being back pain. PEMF therapy offers a safe, non-invasive and drug free approach to pain management and the reduction of pain. It may help reduce pain by promoting the release of endorphins, which are natural pain-relieving substances. It can be a complementary approach for managing chronic pain conditions such as osteoarthritis, fibromyalgia or musculoskeletal injuries. Pain reduction is one of the most common reported benefits of PEMF.

Reduced Inflammation

One of the most commonly reported benefits of PEMF is the reduction of inflammation, which is the precursor of most pain and many different kinds of disorders. The anti-inflammatory effects of PEMF therapy are attributed to several mechanisms:

1. **Enhanced Blood Flow:** PEMF therapy increases microcirculation, which helps to reduce inflammation and swelling by improving the delivery of oxygen and nutrients to the affected areas and enhancing the removal of waste products.

2. **Cellular Repair:** The electromagnetic pulses stimulate cellular repair processes, helping to restore normal cellular function and reduce inflammatory responses.

3. **Modulation of Inflammatory Mediators:** PEMF therapy can influence the production of cytokines and other inflammatory mediators, reducing pro-inflammatory signals and promoting anti-inflammatory responses.

Improved Sleep

PEMF has been shown to improve various kinds of sleep disorders such as insomnia. It also increases overall energy during the day, which coincides with better sleep. Research supports the efficacy of PEMF therapy in improving sleep quality, showing that it can be a beneficial non-invasive treatment for those experiencing sleep disorders or disruptions. By addressing underlying issues such as pain, stress, and hormonal imbalances, PEMF therapy offers a holistic approach to enhancing sleep.

Increased Range of Motion

Muscles, tendons and ligaments relax and loosen up after a PEMF treatment. Many professional athletes use PEMF pre and post workout or competitions. Increased flexibility or movement is one of the first things many people notice, sometimes after one treatment. Another is a general feeling of relaxation. Some of the time, this is very apparent in the face. The face holds a lot of marking signals. Many times after a treatment, I've seen a significant relaxation or smoothness in a person's face even if they haven't noticed anything themselves. Another advantage of PEMF would be to chiropractors or anyone doing any kind of bodily manipulation. Having a PEMF treatment before the manipulation can really relax the body, which in most cases would improve the overall outcome for the patient.

Faster healing after surgery

PEMF is slowly being used more and more after many kinds of surgery such as open heart and plastic surgery in the US. Patients have been found to heal much faster and bruising disappears two to three times as fast.

Depression & Anxiety

PEMF is FDA approved in the US for depression and anxiety unresponsive to pharmaceuticals. I've had some positive results using PEMF to treat depression, anxiety and PTSD. I devised a treatment protocol for depression at a wellness seminar. It was at a time when the microbiome first became a hot topic. I heard over and over about the importance of the gut/brain connection at the seminar. Most PEMF treatments for depression focus on treating just the head, but it didn't take me very long to realize that the head was only half the treatment. The gut is the obvious other half, which needs a boost in energy besides the brain. There is an intrinsic connection between the gut and the brain, which has received extensive media coverage. That's how the gut/brain PEMF treatment protocol developed. I also use it for autoimmune disorders and a general health supercharge.

Faster healing of skin wounds

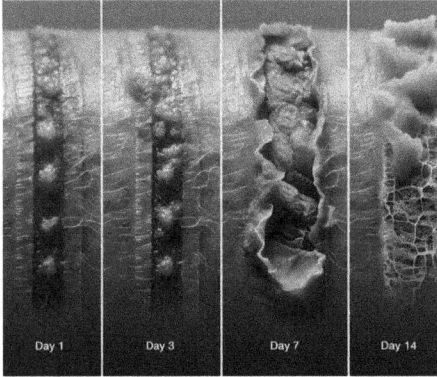

Day 1   Day 3   Day 7   Day 14

Wounds heal faster with PEMF

Over the years, PEMF therapy has been utilized in clinical practice to promote the healing of chronic wounds in both humans and animals. This non-invasive approach has shown very promising results, particularly in cases where wounds have remained unhealed for a significant period of time.

What makes PEMF therapy noteworthy is its ability to target cellular processes involved in wound healing. The electromagnetic fields generated by PEMF devices can penetrate deep into tissues, stimulating cellular activities such as increased production of growth factors, improved blood flow and enhanced tissue regeneration. These effects can promote the healing process and encourage the closure of chronic wounds that have previously resisted other treatments. There is very little contact necessary to treat a wound. Wound dressings do not need to be removed, as electromagnetic waves pass freely through the dressing.

It is particularly remarkable that some chronic wounds, which have persisted for years without improvement, have demonstrated positive responses to PEMF therapy. While the exact mechanisms underlying the benefits of PEMF therapy are still being investigated, the accumulated clinical evidence suggests its potential as a valuable therapeutic option for chronic wound management.

Enhanced Capillary Formation

Studies have demonstrated that PEMF treatment can enhance capillary density and promote new cellular growth (angiogenesis), leading to improved oxygen delivery and facilitating the healing process.

Accelerated Nerve Regeneration

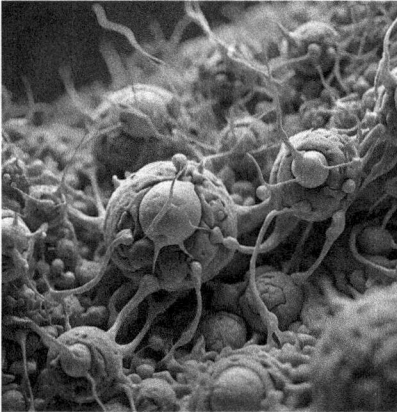

NASA did a landmark study in 2003-2007 on PEMF where it found that a low frequency and low intensity square wave improved circulation, reduced inflammation and enhanced tissue repair. The NASA study also found a 250% to 400% increase in neurogenesis or the formation of neurons. It also showed the stimulation of growth and differentiation of stem cells.

Neurological problems are notoriously slow to heal as a general rule. I've had two people with post-concussion syndrome or TBI (traumatic brain injury) where they were both in accidents and ended up with a concussion that never went away. One had it ongoing for ten years and the other for thirteen years. Both had their symptoms slowly disappear and melt away using the gut/brain treatment protocol after two to three months of using the system twice a day. Two health practitioners treating one of the patients were so impressed with the results that they purchased PEMF systems for their practice.

Stimulates Reflexology & Acupuncture Points

PEMF therapy has the potential to elicit responses in the body similar to those observed in reflexology and acupuncture. Acupuncture meridians are known to have a bioelectrical nature. PEMF can induce bioelectrical currents throughout the entire body. This has the effect of enhancing the flow and charge within all the meridians simultaneously. Recent research indicates that PEMF therapy can stimulate and activate acupuncture points and meridians, similar to the effects of manual acupuncture, but without the requirement for needles.

Increased Production of Nitric Oxide

Clinical studies have demonstrated that PEMF therapy can enhance the release of nitric oxide in the body. Nitric oxide plays a crucial role in signaling and also dilating blood vessels, leading to a reduction in blood pressure, particularly in individuals with hypertension. Additionally, PEMF has been shown to decrease blood viscosity, further contributing to the lowering of blood pressure. The increase in nitric oxide levels induced by PEMF therapy not only improves circulation and oxygenation but also promotes the release of antioxidants within the body. As a result, the presence of antioxidants helps reduce the levels of harmful free radicals, which can have damaging effects on cells and tissues.

Improved Microcirculation

PEMF therapy has been observed to have several effects on the circulatory system that contribute to improved microcirculation, enhanced oxygenation, improved nutrient delivery to tissues and an overall increase in energy. These effects include dilation of capillaries, thinning the viscosity of the blood along with reducing blood pressure. PEMF also inhibits the clumping of red blood cells, known as the Rouleaux effect or agglutination, which can impede proper circulation.

Individuals who have undergone live blood analysis before and after PEMF treatment see noticeable changes in their blood. Apart from observing the separation of red blood cells due to reduced clumping, one prominent observation is the increased speed of blood flow. This heightened flow indicates improved microcirculation, which can contribute to a feeling of increased energy.

Increased Supply of Oxygen, ATP production, Ions and Nutrients

The increased cellular metabolism stimulated by PEMF therapy enhances the efficiency of cellular processes. Cells become more receptive to the absorption of nutrients, allowing for improved uptake of essential nutrients necessary for their proper functioning. Simultaneously, the transfer of ions and electrical signals across cell membranes through voltage-gated ion channels and gap junctions becomes more efficient, facilitating optimal cellular communication, signaling and function.

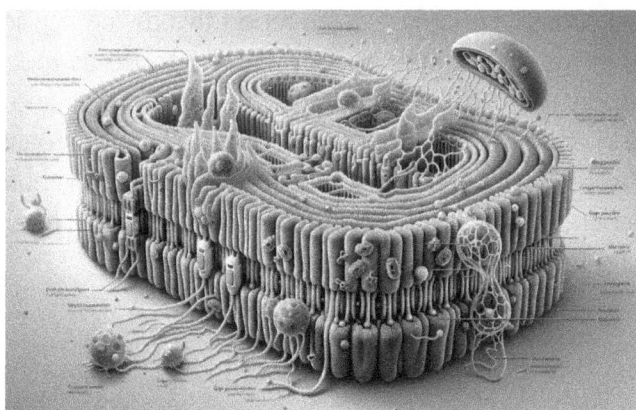

Mitochondria, gap junctions & voltage-gated ion channels

Furthermore, PEMF therapy supports better oxygenation of tissues. By increasing circulation and blood flow, more oxygen is delivered to the cells. Oxygen plays a crucial role in cellular respiration, specifically within the mitochondria. The mitochondria utilize oxygen in the process of ATP production through oxidative phosphorylation. ATP is the primary energy fuel of cells, providing the energy needed for various cellular functions and processes.

With enhanced oxygen supply and circulation, the mitochondria have the necessary resources to produce ATP more effectively. This translates into increased cellular energy levels, which can contribute to improved overall functioning and vitality.

The effects of PEMF therapy can vary significantly between individuals both in the degree of response and on the timing of any positive response. Everyone is different. The specific mechanisms through which PEMF influences cellular efficiency and ATP production are still under study.

Increased Energy

One of the most frequently reported benefits of PEMF therapy is an increased sense of energy. People report this as feeling 'lighter' or they say things don't physically or mentally require as much effort. Some report that life feels smoother. Dovetailed with the general increase in energy can be reports of mental clarity, decreased brain fog and a feeling of not being so mentally or emotionally burdened. I had one person tell me that their decision making was much easier after doing PEMF.

Stronger Bones

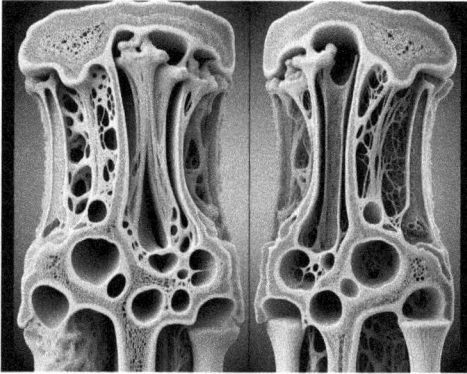

PEMF is FDA approved for bone fractures that won't heal (non-union fractures). It has also been clinically proven to increase bone density, cartilage growth and bone regeneration. I've I have two female clients in their seventies who have been using PEMF for several years. Recently, both had bone density scans showing an increase in bone density, which is quite unusual. Typically, bone density decreases by around 5% annually.

Increased Collagen Production

Collagen is a crucial protein that provides structural support and strength to various tissues in the body, including the skin, tendons, ligaments and bones. As we age, collagen production naturally declines, leading to signs of aging such as wrinkles, sagging skin with reduced elasticity.

Clinical studies investigating the effects of PEMF therapy have shown positive outcomes in terms of collagen production. PEMF treatments have been observed to stimulate the production of collagen in the body, promoting tissue repair and rejuvenation. This increase in collagen synthesis can result in improved skin texture, firmness and overall anti-aging benefits.

Due to the promising findings from these studies, many anti-aging centers and aesthetic clinics have started incorporating PEMF therapy into their treatment protocols. The use of PEMF technology offers a non-invasive and potentially effective approach to address collagen loss and promote a more youthful appearance.

Promotes Bone, Cartilage, Tendon & Soft Tissue Growth

PEMF therapy has shown very promising results in promoting the growth and repair of various musculoskeletal tissues, including bones, cartilage, tendons and soft tissues. In the case of bone growth, PEMF therapy has been studied for its potential to enhance bone formation and accelerate the healing of fractures. Research shows that PEMF can significantly stimulate osteoblast growth. Osteoblasts are the cells responsible for bone formation, leading to increased bone density and improved healing outcomes.

When it comes to cartilage, PEMF therapy has demonstrated positive effects on cartilage repair and regeneration. Studies have shown that PEMF can stimulate chondrocytes, the cells found in cartilage, to enhance the production of extracellular matrix components and promote cartilage healing in conditions such as osteoarthritis.

Tendon and soft tissue healing can also be facilitated by PEMF therapy. Studies have indicated that PEMF can promote the proliferation and alignment of tenocytes, the cells responsible for tendon tissue, leading to improved tendon healing and regeneration.

Anti-Aging

PEMF (Pulsed Electromagnetic Field) therapy has garnered attention in the realm of anti-aging due to its potential effects on cellular rejuvenation, tissue repair and overall well-being. While research on the specific anti-aging benefits of PEMF is still evolving, some findings suggest its potential as a complementary approach in combating certain aspects of aging.

One key aspect of aging is the decline in cellular voltage, functionality and energy production. The observed increase in cellular metabolism and ATP production by PEMF may help mitigate some of the effects associated with cellular aging and support overall vitality.

PEMF therapy also has the potential to influence oxidative stress and inflammation, both of which play significant roles in the aging process. Studies have shown that PEMF may help regulate oxidative stress markers and modulate inflammatory responses. This promotes a balanced environment that can aid in slowing down age-related degenerative processes.

Cell Voltage and Aging

We use PEMF to charge the cells in the body to address any low voltage area in the body due to chronic conditions or injuries. We also need to address the process of aging. An essential point for every individual to note is that as you grow older, your cellular voltage gradually decreases. Therefore, because voltage directly affects how fast the body heals, it's going to take longer to recover or heal as we age.

The following research gives a good snapshot of one role of the electrome, which in essence, is the body's bioelectrical network. The electrome is defined as a novel term for the totality of all the non-neural (excluding the nervous system) currents of a living entity... what I would call the bio-electromagnetic operating system of the body.

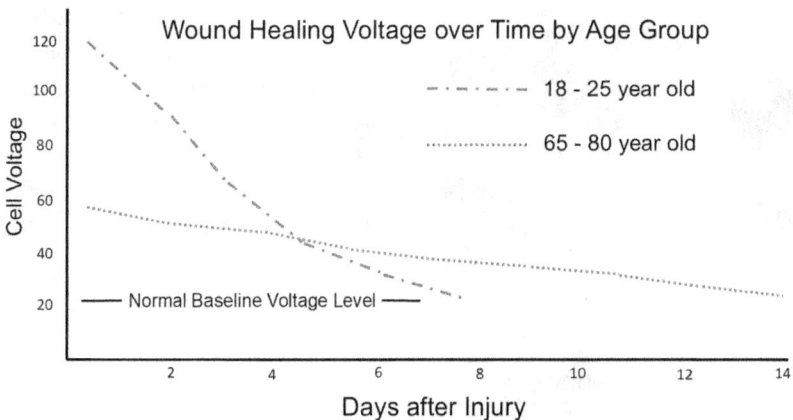

Wound Healing Voltage over Time by Age Group

— · — · — · — 18 - 25 year old

················ 65 - 80 year old

—— Normal Baseline Voltage Level ——

Cell Voltage

Days after Injury

As mentioned previously, Richard Nuccitelli invented the Dermacorder in 2011, which could measure the voltage around a wound. Nuccitelli found a direct correlation between the intensity of the wound's voltage and the timely progression of the healing process. The voltage of the wound peaks the highest at the very time of the injury and slowly decreases as the wound heals over time. It eventually returns to a baseline level of the surrounding tissue voltage when the wound has fully healed. Nuccitelli discovered that people with a higher peak voltage healed quicker that those that had a lower voltage throughout the healing process. This increase in voltage was measured and it was found that an eighteen to twenty-five-year-old had over double the cellular voltage surrounding a wound as a sixty-five-year-old to eighty-year-old. This is one of the principal reasons things take longer to heal as you get older. As we age, our cellular voltage decreases and that alone is a fundamental reason to consider adopting PEMF.

"The basis of life is bioelectric. We are electric beings." – Richard Nuccitelli

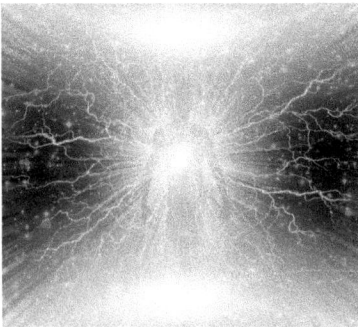

This is clear evidence of the importance of maintaining or even increasing your cellular voltage, which governs much of the overall efficiency of the biochemistry of the body as detailed above.

Cellular voltage or your bioelectric potential governs:

1. The speed of your recovery
2. The efficiency of your metabolism

3. Cellular communication

4. New cell development and growth

5. Stem cell proliferation

6. Osmosis through cell membranes

7. Cell respiration and detoxification

8. Blood circulation efficiency

9. Your overall level of energy, which can be felt

Besides the metaphor of your cells being similar to a battery, your bioelectrical potential or the whole bioelectrical network of the body is very comparable to the operating system of a computer. A computer operating system is defined as the basic software program that acts as an interface between the computer (in this example - your body) and the computer hardware (your brain, organs, genetic code (DNA), etc.

Electromagnetic radiation is the fundamental form of information in nature and one of the four fundamental forces of nature. These electromagnetic signals are the language or software through which atoms and molecules communicate and the method by which organisms also receive information from their surrounding environment.

The bioelectrical intelligence or software ultimately controls the operation of many bodily functions and programs that can directly impact the state of your health. If the operating system (your bioelectrical system) is sluggish or inefficient due to an insufficient reserve of energy (low cellular voltage) then many things in regards to your health can be affected. This can result in a slow or sluggish immune system, lethargic metabolism and low energy. It can also reside at a level that is below the threshold for the immune system to be able to make a significant or effective healing response. Again, it's comparable to a flat car battery with not enough energy to run things efficiently or sometimes even start the car.

Increased Absorption of Nutrients

PEMF therapy has shown its potential to enhance the absorption of nutrients in the body. There are some indications that PEMF therapy may have positive effects on nutrient uptake and utilization. One proposed mechanism is the influence of PEMF therapy on cellular membrane permeability. It has been suggested that PEMF helps to optimize the functioning of cell membranes, which are responsible for the passage of nutrients into cells. By enhancing the fluidity and permeability of cell membranes and increasing the efficiency of voltage-gated ion channels in the cell membrane, PEMF therapy may facilitate the absorption of essential nutrients.

Additionally, as mentioned before, PEMF therapy has been associated with improved blood flow and circulation. Efficient blood circulation is essential for the transport of nutrients throughout the body. By enhancing blood flow, PEMF therapy may contribute to better nutrient delivery to cells and tissues, thereby supporting optimal absorption and utilization.

Mental Clarity

PEMF therapy has been explored for its potential effects on mental clarity and cognitive function. While research in this area is ongoing and still very limited, there are some indications that PEMF therapy may contribute to improved mental clarity and focus. Personally, I've had many reports of improved mental clarity or a decrease of brain fog from people I've treated or who have rented or purchased a system.

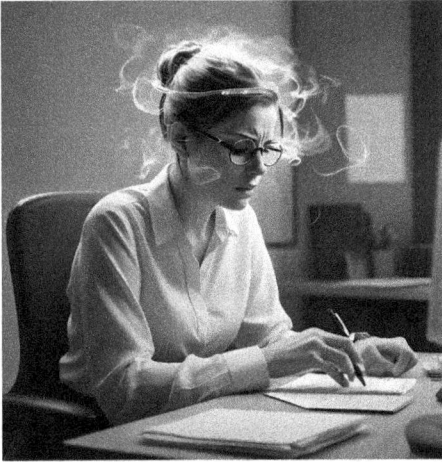

One proposed mechanism is the impact of PEMF therapy on brain activity and neurotransmitter levels. Studies have suggested that PEMF may modulate brain wave patterns, potentially promoting a more balanced and focused state of mind. Additionally, PEMF therapy has been shown to influence the release of certain neurotransmitters, such as dopamine and serotonin, which play crucial roles in mood regulation, cognition and mental well-being.

Another way PEMF therapy may enhance mental clarity is by reducing stress and promoting relaxation. Chronic stress can impair cognitive function and contribute to mental fatigue and brain fog. PEMF therapy has been studied for its potential to modulate stress responses and promote a sense of calm, potentially leading to improved mental clarity and concentration. rTMS (repetitive transcranial magnetic stimulation, which is a form of PEMF is FDA approved in the US and TGA approved in Australia for depression and anxiety.

Furthermore, PEMF therapy has been found to have positive effects on sleep quality. Quality sleep is vital for cognitive function and mental clarity. By improving sleep patterns and promoting deep, restorative sleep, PEMF therapy may indirectly contribute to enhanced mental clarity during waking hours.

Non-Invasive and Well-Tolerated

Low intensity and low frequency PEMF therapy is widely regarded as a safe and non-invasive treatment option, provided that it is used within appropriate parameters. It is generally well tolerated by most individuals and side effects are uncommon, but it can detox the body (see chapter 6).

Detoxification is good sign of a positive response by the body to the PEMF. But it must be done gradually while the body is acclimating to the increased cellular efficiency, which releases metabolic wastes quicker. Detoxing may manifest as lower energy or people feeling that they might be coming down with a slight cold or the flu. This makes PEMF therapy an appealing complement to existing health practices, as it offers additional treatment options with a relatively low risk.

The non-invasive nature of PEMF therapy means that it does not require any surgical procedures or invasive interventions, reducing the potential for complications or adverse reactions. It typically involves the application of electromagnetic fields to specific areas of the body or the entire body, depending on the treatment approach.

Moreover, the well-tolerated nature of PEMF therapy means that most individuals can undergo treatments without experiencing significant discomfort or adverse effects. While individual responses may vary, the majority of people find PEMF therapy to be comfortable and without any notable side effects.

CHAPTER 4

PEMF Therapy Procedures & Treatment Protocols

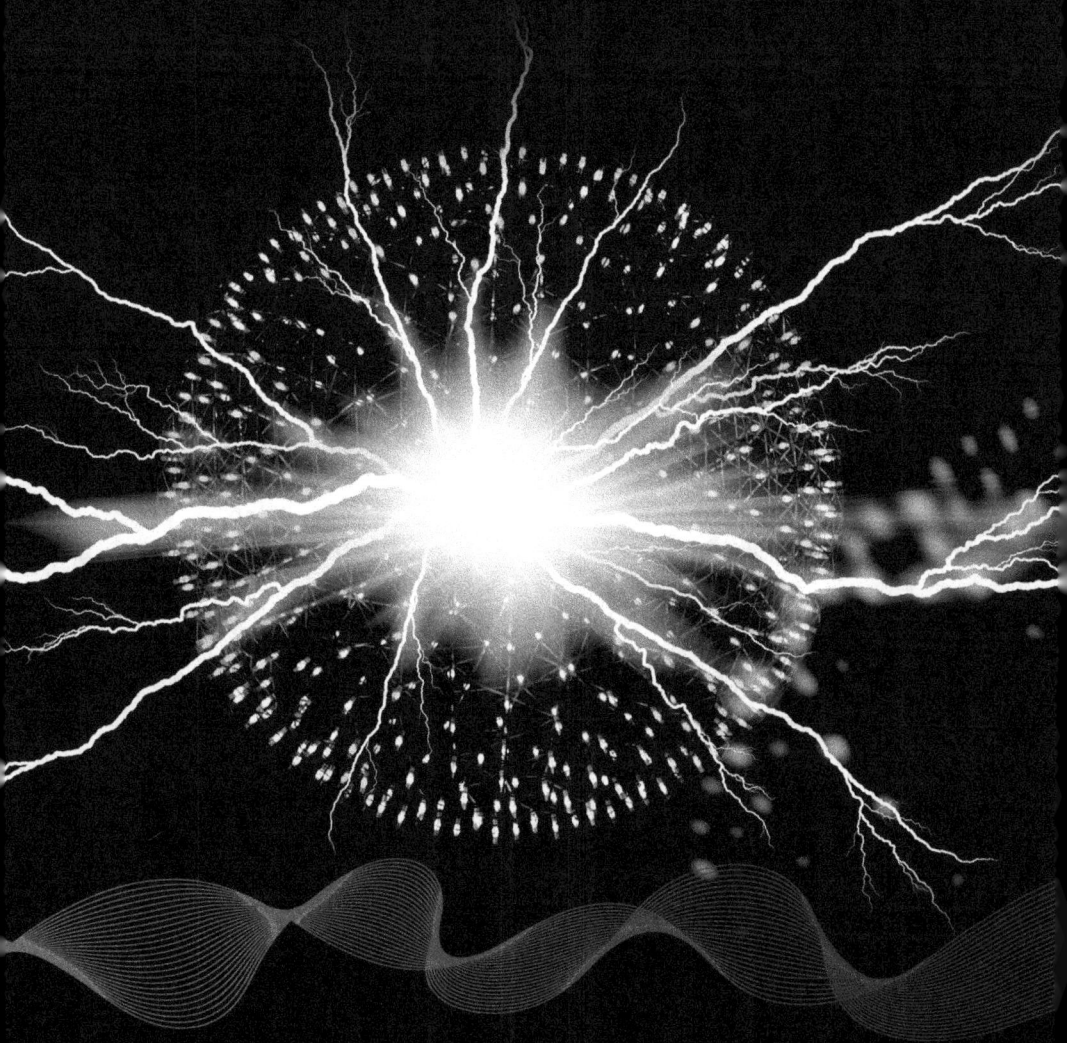

CHAPTER 4
PEMF Therapy Procedures & Treatment Protocols

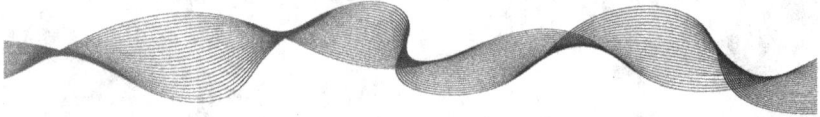

Contraindications -
Specific Conditions When PEMF Should Not Be Used

The contraindications for PEMF:

1 - pregnancy

2 - epilepsy

3 - battery operated devices like pacemakers

4 - anyone with an organ transplant

PEMF should only be used with the approval of a licensed health care professional for someone under medical supervision with the following conditions:

- Presence of tumors

- Serious cardiac arrhythmia

- Acute attacks of hyperthyroidism

- Extreme sensitivity to electromagnetic radiation

Applying PEMF

You don't need to be an expert in physics to learn how to use a PEMF system. The concept of PEMF and the treatments are easy to learn, but it will take a little bit of practice. PEMF is basically a cellular charging system. If you keep this in mind and use this concept when talking about PEMF, then other people will be more likely to understand and more amenable to trying it. This increases the potential for a positive outcome.

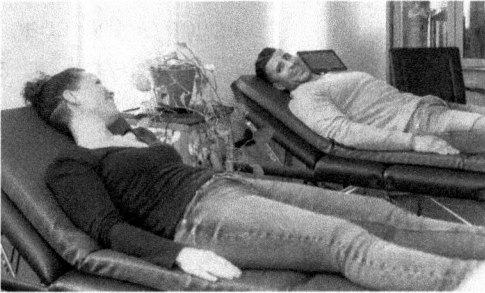

You also need to learn about the hardware in regard to the features and functionalities of the PEMF system. It's very easy to use because it automatically leads you through the settings. Most people are comfortable using the hardware in only fifteen to twenty minutes. That's how easy it is to use. There are also over twenty short two-to-three-minute videos explaining every one of the features and functionalities of the system.

People may ask questions about PEMF or the system, therefore it's good to have some information on hand that you can refer to or even give them. All this is part of the information and training I offer.

Preparing for PEMF Treatments

A PEMF system with a whole-body mat and other applicators requires some space. It's important that the system is freely available for anyone to go on it at any time rather than having to set it up each time. A massage table with a tilt up head section is ideal.

Using a spare bedroom or another free space would also work. It's important to put the whole-body mat on a firm surface. The floor, a firm bed or a couch are alternatives. Caution should be used with a bed or couch. If the mattress is too soft or a person is too heavy, then the copper coils in the full-body mat can be bent or broken. If a bed is used, I highly suggest a piece of plywood or MDF to put under the mat so it doesn't bend or flex too much.

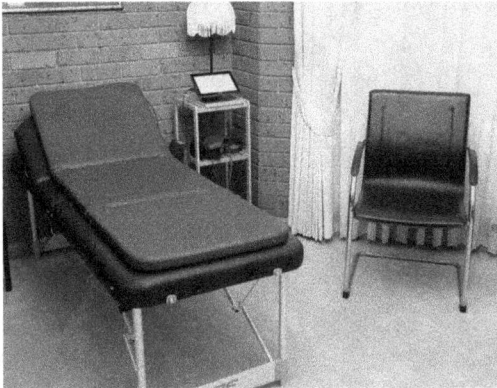

The picture to the left shows an ideal footprint of the space that's required. Find a small stand to put the controller on along with a solid-backed chair. Some parts of the treatment can be done while sitting in the chair. A towel or blanket may come in handy to place under or over a person lying on the mat. The PEMFs pass freely through material of all kinds.

The PEMF system I use is very user friendly and therefore easy to master the control unit with the touchscreen prompting you what to do next. You set time in minutes and one of eight different intensities. There is also a built-in guide (iGuide) listing nearly 300 disorders that gives suggested time and intensity settings for each one of the three applicators. When you first start out, all you have to do is follow the standard treatment protocols. With a little bit of practice, you will become comfortable and it will be second nature to you.

Treatment Protocols

Everyone begins with the same treatment duration and intensity on the whole-body mat. Low and slow is the rule of thumb when first starting out with PEMF. The body needs to acclimate to or adjust to the increase in cellular efficiency created by the PEMF. Much more on this later in Chapter 6.

With the system I use, all that's necessary is to set the time (in minutes) and the intensity on a digital screen. The frequency spectrum or the biological window of resonance is automatically set by the time of day. The focus or range of the frequency spectrum can be manually tweaked if so desired.

Lower time and intensity adjustments may be necessary for individuals who are sensitive. I always ask a person if they're sensitive before any treatment. Sensitive people know they are sensitive. If they are, I'll turn down the intensity to the lowest level or one notch above it.

Applicator Care & Considerations

The PEMF system I use is shown on the right. There is a touchscreen controller with three applicators, which emit the PEMFs. The applicators are the whole-body mat, a pad the size of a pillow and the spot. The spot, which has two palm-size pads that can be wrapped around knees, arms, ankles or laid flat on the body. PEMFs come out both sides of every one of the applicators, therefore it doesn't matter which way you turn them against the body. There's only one exception, which is the whole-body mat that generates far infrared. PEMF comes out on both sides, but the far infrared is only emitted on one side of the mat. You can lie on your back, tummy or side; it doesn't matter. The closer any part of the body is to the mat, pad or spot, then the stronger the electromagnetic field.

PEMF System with Optional Brain Entrainment and Biofeedback Systems

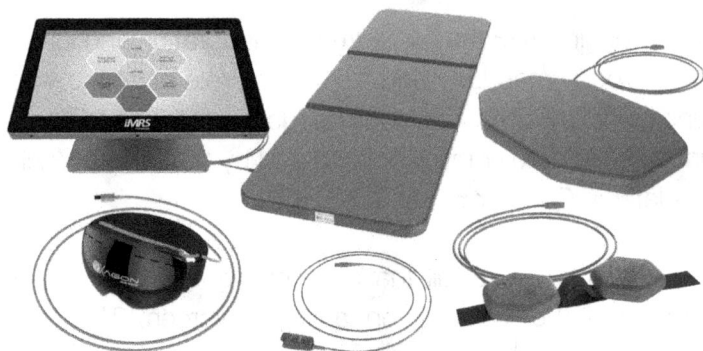

Complete PEMF system with optional brain entrainment & biofeedback systems

The medical-grade vinyl on the applicators can be cleaned with soap and water. You can also cover the full-body mat or other applicators with a towel or sheet if you like. The electromagnetic waves are not affected at all by clothing. The PEMFs pass completely through with no effect on properties of the waves. Metal such as keys, smart phones and wallets should be removed. Major pieces of jewelry and watches should also be taken off. I don't personally worry about pierced earrings, rings or any small jewelry, but a purist might. It's up to you.

People ask if they should sleep on the mat to get better or quicker results. There's no need. PEMF is a cellular charging system like the charger for your smart phone's battery. You can leave your phone plugged into the charger overnight, but the battery is only going to be charged up to 100% and then it stops charging. It's the same with your body. Once the cells are charged, there's no need to continue. It only takes around fifteen minutes on the mat to charge the healthy cells followed by fifteen to twenty minutes using the local applicators on the areas of imbalance or low voltage.

Also, like your smart phone, the charge in your cells will decrease in four to six hours. Renting or purchasing a system allows you to charge yourself a couple of times a day. This enables you to keep your cellular efficiency at a consistently higher threshold of efficiency.

Comprehensive Healing: The Full-Body PEMF Approach

PEMF applicators are what produce the electromagnetic waves, which emanate from the tightly wound copper coils sandwiched between foam and covered with medical grade vinyl. Many high intensity systems don't provide full-body mats but offer hand-held pads, paddles, single loop coils, double loop coils and rope coils.

I believe it's very important to use a whole-body mat that treats every cell in the body all at the same time. This addresses the body as one complete integrated organism to enhance the function of the whole bioelectrical communication system.

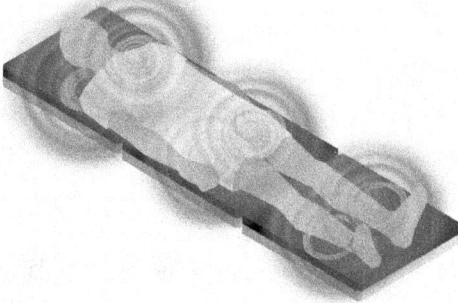

Key reasons to use a whole-body mat:

1 – Western medicine often takes a reductionist approach, which fixates on the health problem where it locally manifests in the body and only treats the localized area *to reduce the symptoms*. There can be other imbalances caused by deficiencies or excesses that are contributing factors to the problem area, which may be located in other parts of the body.

One of the major things I treat with PEMF is the gut microbiome. Imbalances within the gut can impact the health and functionality of the brain. This can have an effect on the immune system, hormone and enzyme production, sleep, stress reactivity, memory, pain sensitivity and a whole slew of other things. Where and how a condition manifests may be the result of a domino or cascading effect as a result of other systems, organs or glands being imbalanced. The area where any imbalance manifests may also create or trigger other imbalances somewhere else in the body. The other imbalances may or may not have manifested yet. Everything is connected, especially bioelectrically, so treating the whole body with a full-body mat is very important and essential in my book (pun intended).

2 – It's beneficial to 'charge' the whole body all at once to establish better cellular communication with all biological systems to assist in delivering a more balanced and efficient physiology. This can help to decrease the probability of any signaling or communication that may be getting blocked or interrupted. You want all systems up and running efficiently along with the best internal communication. Most of the communication is bioelectrical along with the biochemical communication that's traditionally treated with pharmaceuticals. The human body relies on both bioelectrical and biochemical processes for communication and functionality. The distinction between these systems is not absolute, as biochemical processes often influence bioelectrical activity and vice versa.

The nervous system, comprising the central nervous system (brain and spinal cord) and the peripheral nervous system, serves as the major overall operating and communication system in the body. It plays a crucial role in integrating and coordinating both biochemical and bioelectrical signals to maintain homeostasis or balance. The endocrine system, which includes glands that secrete hormones into the bloodstream, also plays a significant role in communication and coordination.

In essence, the nervous and endocrine systems work together to regulate and coordinate the body's functions. These systems integrate bioelectrical and biochemical signaling to ensure the proper functioning of various organs, tissues and cells. While both communication systems are vital, the nervous system is often considered the master regulator due to its rapid signaling capabilities and its role in orchestrating complex physiological responses.

3 – Initially it's important to get the body accustomed to electromagnetic waves and gradually condition the cells to this new experience of increased electromagnetic energy and efficiency. This can be especially important when you use more focused and higher intensity applicators on specific areas of the body. It's also part of the protocols of acclimation for detoxification where you introduce PEMF in a low and slow manner. This is important so the body can gradually adjust and doesn't detox too fast.

4 – The whole-body mat generates an electromagnetic field that completely surrounds and radiates out beyond the surface of the body. Therefore, besides treating the physical body, the whole-body mat also encompasses some of the outer human biofield, which is also electromagnetic. Some people or cultures may call this the human aura or energy field.

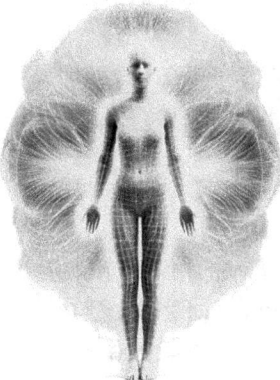

The biofield is an electromagnetic field that surrounds the body. It is very real and has been scientifically measured by a SQUID (superconducting quantum interference device) magnetometer to extend out one to two meters from the body. Ancient cultures have known of its existence for thousands of years. Eileen Day McKusick, who wrote

'Electric Body, Electric Health,' writes extensively about the biofield along with some other notable authors and researchers. What manifests in the body is reflected in the biofield and vice-versa.

"To both understand and treat the entire human being, current practices in Western medicine must expand concepts of healing to incorporate physics of the human energy field (HEF) into modern medical practice. Knowledge of the existence of and effects on the HEF will determine the future of medicine by opening new medical paradigms, integrating Western medicine with Eastern medical practices that have been time tested for thousands of years."

- Christina L Ross, PhD, BCPP Wake Forest Center for Integrative Medicine.

Whole-body mat Treatment

I always begin a PEMF treatment session with the whole-body mat, usually for 10 to 15 minutes at an intensity of 25 or 50 on my PEMF system. This intensity is at the lower range of the system. I do this because there's one side effect that you need to be careful of and that's detoxification: see Chapter 6. Some people may have difficulty with lying flat on the full-body mat. A small pillow or rolled towel under the neck or knees can help support the body to make them more comfortable.

The whole-body mat generates pre-programmed frequency patterns. Based on the time of the day, it shifts the focus of the frequency spectrum into four different segments (morning, noon, evening and night). This is achieved by delivering higher beta frequencies in the morning to energize you. In the evening you get the lower and relaxing delta and theta frequencies automatically. The time variance of the frequencies delivered is based on the naturally observed circadian rhythms. Circadian rhythms have been scientifically proven with a Nobel Prize given in 2017 to Hall, Rosbash and Young for their research.

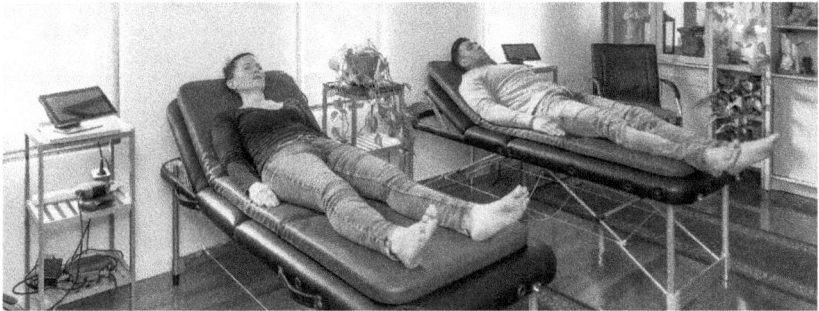

Since frequencies are automatically adjusted, the only two variables that need to be set are intensity and time. The most effective way to gauge PEMF treatment results is to adjust only one factor, which is the intensity. Otherwise, if you change both time and intensity and things change for the better or worse, then you need to know what variable was responsible for the noted difference. If you change both, then it's very difficult to tell what factor was responsible for the noted effect. Was it the time, the intensity or both? You can't tell at all.

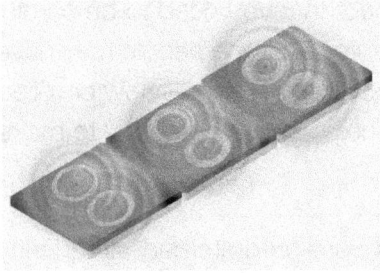

The whole-body mat has six large copper coils the size of dinner plates that generate a triple sawtooth waveform. This waveform is very effective in inducting microcurrents in the cells. It also creates numerous frequencies that fall within the biological window of resonance to harmonize with all the different cellular frequencies of the body.

The most effective waveforms have a steep rise and fall like the square wave and the triple sawtooth. These waveforms are very effective in inducing microcurrents in the cells. A sine wave is far less effective in inducing microcurrents in the cells because of the gradual rise and fall of the waveform. The sine wave is commonly found in cheaper PEMF systems because it is easy and inexpensive to generate and does not require a sophisticated signal generator.

Localized Applicator Treatment

After using the full-body mat for ten to fifteen minutes, I immediately follow it with the localized applicators for ten to twenty minutes. There are also copper coils in the local applicators (pad and spot), which generate square waves. The square wave is sometimes called the NASA wave. NASA, the National Aeronautics and Space Administration in the US, did a four-year study on PEMF from 2003 to 2007. They employed a square wave at 10Hz in the same intensity range of the system I use. One result of the NASA study was a 250% to 400% increase in neural stem cell growth.

Some systems offer a dual mode functionality where you can run two applicators at the same time. For example, one person can be lying on the full-body mat while another person can be using the pad or spot on a problem area. Or one person could be using the pad on the chest or back, while at the same time, using the spot to treat a knee or ankle. The localized applicators can be placed on top or under the body while either lying down or sitting in a chair. This a great time saver.

One thing you don't want to do is to lie on the full-body mat getting a treatment, while at the same time, using the pad or the spot. In this case, PEMFs are coming up through the body from the mat and also going down through the body from one of the localized applicators. Therefore, we have waves intersecting like ripples of water meeting. This creates constructive or destructive wave interference patterns. In other words, the waves can cancel each other out or become distorted.

The pad and the spot both generate a square wave, which is different than the full-body mat (sawtooth wave). What's important to note is that it's not redundant to use the mat immediately followed by the local applicators because of the use of two different waveforms. This is one of the unique features of the system I use. It's the combination of the two unique waveforms that I see the best results.

I've seen people receive very positive results with their PEMF systems using the mat and the localized applicators. Upon reconnecting years later, some people have informed me that their condition had stagnated or even deteriorated. Upon checking their treatment protocols, I found that many have taken 'shortcuts' to save time. They either laid on the full-body mat and don't use the local applicators or only used the local applicators without the full-body mat. Once they resumed doing both the mat and the local applicators, then things improved again.

The pad and spot don't use the principle of the circadian rhythms like the full-body mat. They deliver a full spectrum of frequencies within the biological window of resonance. The pad and the spot are more focused PEMF applicators to address specific targeted areas where an imbalance appears in the body. These problem areas are what I term low voltage areas of imbalance. In this scenario, one of the contributing factors can be a deficit in cellular voltage or a blockage of voltage to the area. This low voltage threshold may be insufficient to maintain or repair the cells and tissues in that area.

A low voltage threshold can be one of the contributing factors or deficits associated with a chronic condition or injury. The level of cellular voltage is an important factor that governs the degree of efficiency and level of communication of many other systems in the body. As stated previously, it's very comparable to the operating system of a computer, which is what Michael Levin of Tufts University calls the non-neural bioelectrical system of the body.

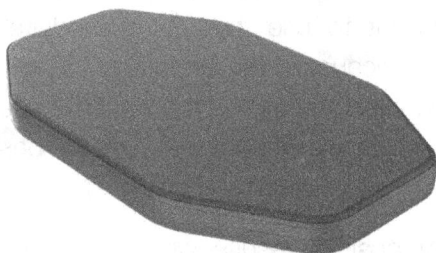

I use the pad for less localized areas of the body like the thoracic area, the back, across the shoulders, the feet, knees and hips. A problematic issue like a painful shoulder is associated with a low voltage or a blockage or disrupted energy flow. Other factors may be contributing to the problem such as an injury, inflammation, nerve damage, etc. The low voltage in the shoulder can drain energy from the rest of the body. People often describe the effects of pain as sapping their energy, which can be attributed to a loss or a blockage of electron flow in the affected area.

When treating a problem on one side of the body, it's best to address both sides simultaneously. The seemingly unaffected side may be under additional stress by compensating for the imbalance on the troublesome side. For example, a problem in the right foot could potentially stress the left foot as the body tries to maintain balance.

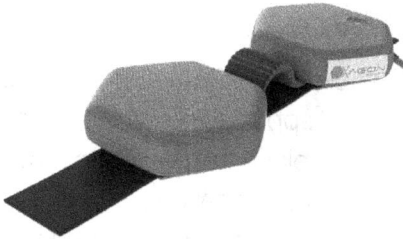

A good treatment protocol is to place the pad on the floor, sit in a chair and put both feet on the pad. Don't directly stand on it, but put each foot in the center of each half. Some people who can't feel anything while lying on the mat can feel the energy of the PEMF shooting up their legs. The PEMF comes out equally on both sides of the mat, pad and spot.

While the pad and the spot both produce a square wave, the spot applicator has its own unique property. The difference between the spot and the pad is intensity and area of coverage. The spot applicator has more copper windings in it, therefore it generates a magnetic field four times stronger than the mat or the pad at the same intensity setting. The spot is for more concentrated and localized application of PEMFs to a smaller area. The two palm-sized pads of the spot are connected by a band of elastic on one side and Velcro on the other. It can be wrapped around ankles, knees, elbows or draped over a shoulder. It can also lie flat on any part of the body. I've used it on breasts, ovaries, the prostrate, jaws, the spine, the neck, head, ears etc.

The other unique feature of the spot is that you can sandwich a body part like a knee with the two pads on opposite sides of the knee and parallel to each other. The two pads are wired in series, which when placed parallel to each other creates what is called a Helmholtz coil arrangement or Helmholtz effect. This is where the magnetic field strength is relatively uniform all the way through the body. Normally the magnetic field strength diminishes the further the distance from the copper coils.

Local Applicator Positioning

People ask where to put the local applicators. Common sense for most issues will tell you to place the local applicators over a problem area. If you have a bad knee or back, just place the pad or spot over or under the problem area. The positioning of local applicators (pad and spot) varies depending on the specific health issue along with the time and intensity, a topic I cover in the training after a system is purchased.

With issues like depression, autoimmune or neurological conditions, I suggest doing the gut/brain treatment protocol. Start out with the full-body mat for the prescribed time. Then immediately follow with the pad on the lower abdomen and the spot lying flat behind the head with the other little pad next to it behind the neck. Of course, the pad and the spot can be used at the same time if you have the split mode option on your system that allows two applicators to be used at the same time.

Using the mat followed by the local applicator(s) is considered one treatment session. I suggest to do this twice a day if you have a system. One treatment session or the actual cellular charge will last around six hours more or less. Some individuals experience immediate effects, while others may notice changes later as the cellular charge continues to work over the hours. Others may not notice any differences at all until much later. Healing takes time… this is the nature of the healing process. People also respond differently, especially with respect to time. Some respond nearly immediately and for others it can take a long time.

Those who experience benefits might find these effects lasting for several days. Since results vary from person to person, the only way to truly know is to try it. All you have to look out for is detoxification, but it's important to go slow and easy, especially with the intensity. Detoxification is a good sign that the body is beginning to respond, but you want to do it gradually so the body can expel it thoroughly.

Varying the Intensity

One of my cardinal rules when applying PEMF therapy is to vary the intensity and not set the same level every time for every single treatment. What I like to do is vary the intensity up or down a notch or two for each treatment. This is especially important for those who rent or own PEMF systems and are doing one or two treatments every day over a period of time. The reason for this is due to the body's inherent tendency to acclimate or habituate to any kind of treatment.

The concept of acclimation in the body refers to the physiological adjustments that occur over time in response to consistent exposure to stimuli, such as therapeutic treatments, drugs or exercise. The human body is remarkably adaptable, and as it encounters repetitive or prolonged influences, it tends to develop mechanisms to diminish their effects, even if they are good for the body. This tendency and adaptability of the body is both a strength and a challenge, particularly in the context of therapeutic treatments, drugs and exercise routines.

In the realm of medical treatments, the phenomenon of acclimation can be observed when the body gradually becomes less responsive to a particular therapy or drug. Over time, the efficacy of a drug can diminish as the body adapts to its presence, potentially requiring adjustments to the treatment plan, such as changes in dosage or the introduction of alternative medications.

Similarly, with exercise, the body tends to acclimate to a specific workout routine. Initially, a particular exercise regimen may yield significant benefits, but as the body becomes accustomed to the routine, the gains may plateau or even reverse to a degree. This is why fitness experts often emphasize the importance of incorporating variety into exercise programs to continuously challenge the body and prevent adaptation-induced stagnation. In essence, the body's tendency to acclimate underscores the need for diversity and variation. This is the reason I suggest to vary the intensity up or down a bit if you are doing PEMF on a regular basis.

How Long for PEMF to Work

Many people ask how long it will take to see a result. The simple answer is that there is no way to tell. Some people can experience an improvement on the first treatment... with others it may take months. The timing of a response varies, as each individual reacts in their own unique way. Still, the ratio of positive results is very good relatively speaking. Around eighty percent see a positive result and twenty percent don't see much difference.

Many times, people will notice improvements with other aspects of their health. They may notice more energy, better sleep, improved mental clarity and feeling more relaxed, while the main problem is still lingering around. It's still a good sign that their body is beginning to respond if the little things start falling away first. Other times the main health issue can be the first to respond and improve.

I've had pain levels reduce by a factor of two to five points on a ten-point scale in just one treatment. With others, no effect at all, even after the first treatment or subsequent treatments. Many have taken weeks of treatment before they notice a difference. I've also had people phone me several hours after a treatment to report a significant improvement. This is a good example of the cellular charge continuing to work for four to six hours where it finally kicks in with a positive result.

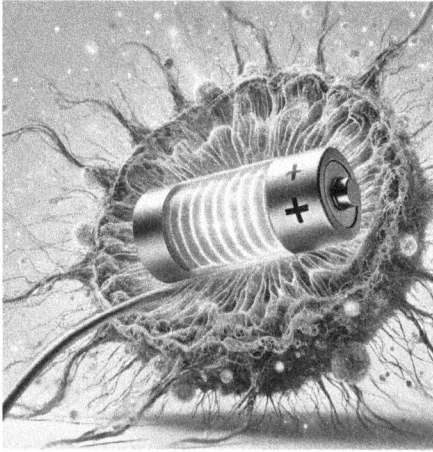

Similar to a battery, the cells will retain the additional charge provided during the treatment for four to six hours. The voltage level then decreases back to their baseline level, which is unique to each individual. This is what I call the charging inertia or a bioelectrical momentum, which still functions after the treatment due to the increased charge that is held in the body. Sometimes, this increased cellular charge and the corresponding improved physiological efficiency takes some time before any positive results manifest with reduced pain, inflammation, swelling, stiffness or improved sleep. As a very general rule-of-thumb, the pain reduction or other benefits can last on average for a couple of days. Of course, for some it can be a shorter time or even a much longer time

Here is a good example: I met a man in his 40s who was in a lot of pain in his joints. He rented a PEMF system for three weeks. He did treatments twice a day every day and nothing happened until near the end of the third week. Then within the third week over one or two days, the pain melted away and was 90% gone. I can only surmise that he reached some kind of threshold where the continuous increased cellular charge finally reached a state where the body could neutralize the pain.

To continue the story, which may also help to answer another question; he then stopped for a week to see what would happen. He called me at the end of the next week to rent the system again because the pain had returned. He rented it one more week and then decided to purchase a system once he saw the pain diminish much sooner. He was a serious weightlifter and would not change his lifestyle and stop lifting weights, so the PEMF served as a solution to his problem, but it didn't cure it.

With questions about how long it takes for PEMF to help, comes an additional question about curing health conditions. As stated at the beginning of the book, PEMF does not cure anything. PEMF therapy boosts cellular voltage potentials and this can contribute to an increase in the biological efficiency of the body to restore or maintain better health. It's usually not just one imbalance in the body like low cellular voltage. Low voltage potential may be one of the contributing factors, but as written previously, there are usually other contributing factors. It's always best to take a holistic approach by looking at nutrition, mental or emotional issues and the state of your gut… your microbiome. There are lots of books on these subjects and I highly recommend for people to take charge of their own health. No one else is going to look after you or care for you any better than yourself.

"All disease begins in the gut."
– Hippocrates

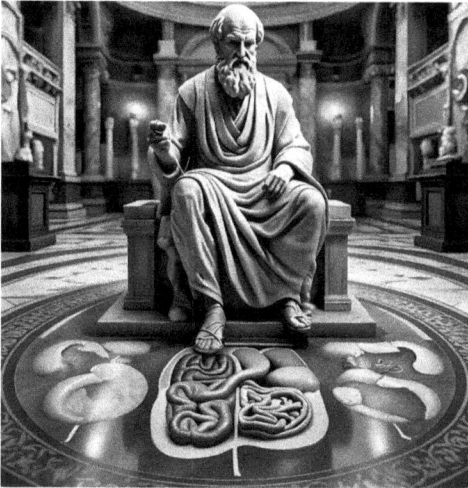

Another question asked is how often should someone have a PEMF treatment. I can only speak from the perspective of using a low intensity PEMF system, which can be used on a daily basis. Many experts using high intensity systems don't advise using their systems every day. One of the many advantages of a low intensity system is that it is safe and also beneficial to use every day. So, knowing that a cellular charge lasts for four to six hours, you *should* do it at least once daily... preferably twice a day if you own or are renting a system. Obviously, most people can't do this if they are visiting a PEMF practitioner for treatments.

Personally, I do two PEMF treatment sessions on the mat and pad/ spot every day and will do this for the rest of my life. I say this for one reason... 'If you'd seen what I've seen PEMF can do for people, then you would get a system and use it for the rest of *your* life, even if there's nothing wrong with you.' I emphasize again, that as you age your cellular voltage declines. Cellular voltage, or your bioelectrical potential, governs a vast majority of many physiological processes in the body. It's like the operating system of a computer or your body's bioelectrical network that's connected to everything in the body. It's the spark of life or your life force. We *are* literally 'electric.'

"The human body is a dynamic, electromagnetic organism, resonating with the frequencies of the environment."

– Dr Richard Gerber

If you don't have a system and you are seeing a practitioner, I'd initially recommend two to three treatments per week. Of course, some people won't be able to manage two to three treatments for various reasons. Some people will still see results in just receiving one treatment per week, but the probability goes up for potential benefits to manifest sooner the more often they attend… especially at first. The more frequent people keep their metabolic and biochemical efficiencies up-and-running at a higher level, the sooner the potential to see positive benefits.

A treatment takes approximately forty-five to sixty minutes depending on the health issues to be addressed. Everyone starts out with the same time and intensity in the initial treatment with some variation for sensitive people. That may change after the first treatment. It's best to go by how the body responds and the feedback from the previous treatment. Everyone reacts differently and at a different pace, which necessitates making changes to time, intensity and possibly treatment intervals. In the end, the body's response is always the best meter to gauge or to 'read' in order to determine the course of action for the next treatment.

Neurological issues are notoriously slow to respond, but I've also had some very good outcomes in a relatively short period of time. That's an exception to the rule. Most likely, we are talking in timeframes of months with many neurological conditions. It's usually best to manage expectations about PEMF from the very beginning. I prefer to be very conservative when estimating time frames or outcomes. Ideally, PEMF will yield positive results much sooner than anticipated. I personally don't like to guess at all. I like to take a wait-and-see approach, but of course I always hope for the best.

Helpful Hints for Practitioners

Treating people is the best way to learn about PEMF and to build confidence. It helps you understand the technology's capabilities, identify areas for improvement and to see the results to share other people's experiences with potential clients.

While some practitioners are cautious about introducing PEMF to their existing clientele, it's important to start treating people as soon as you learn the simple basics. Relying solely on self-treatment or family members may not provide meaningful results, especially if you're asymptomatic. Instead, consider offering free initial treatments to a select few so you can begin to see with your own eyes what you may have been reading about in the literature.

Remember that PEMF doesn't work for everyone, but it has a good success rate and very minimal side effects. Results can vary with some people responding quickly and others requiring consistent application over time.

To become more comfortable with the equipment and treatment protocols, also consider adding an explanation of how PEMF works (found in the following section). If you explain how PEMF works in straightforward, easy-to-understand terms, this helps create a positive mental framework for your clients and establishes a deeper connection. Remember, PEMF is completely new to most people, so providing clear guidance helps them feel more comfortable and receptive to the treatment. Your ability to communicate the therapy authentically on one level shows that you care about your clients' health.

It's also important to recognize that a positive inner belief, or the placebo effect, can play a significant role in the healing process. Bruce Lipton, author of "The Biology of Belief," suggests that the placebo effect can account for up to 30% of a treatment's effectiveness. Embrace this aspect of healing, as it can enhance the overall results of PEMF or any other therapy. I hope these suggestions will help you gain experience, build confidence and improve your ability to help clients with PEMF therapy.

'The natural healing force within each of us is the greatest force in getting well. Healing is a matter of time, but it is sometimes also a matter of opportunity.' – Hippocrates

Information Shared During a Treatment

When commencing a treatment, I like to convey the following:

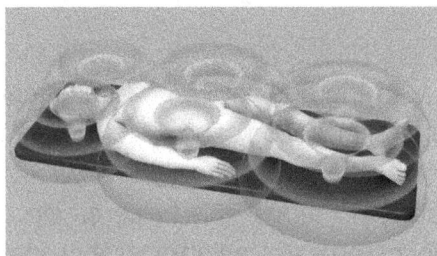

The whole-body mat you're lying on has large copper coils in it. When an electric current is passed through a copper coil, it generates an electromagnetic field; that's basic physics.

Electromagnetic fields are unique; they go completely through your body and clothing. So, in effect, your whole body is being bathed in a natural electromagnetic cloud. This cloud is pulsing on and off at the same rate that matches the same frequency and the same voltage of your cells. Every cell, tissue and organ in your body is being treated all at once by the natural pulsating waves.

Not many therapies reach every cell in the body all at once. Most people don't feel anything with a low intensity system. Some may feel a slight tingling in different parts of the body while others may feel some heat due to the increase in circulation.

The electromagnetic field is actually passing through every cell in the body while we simultaneously pulse the field by switching it on and off. When pulsed electromagnetic waves are turned on and off, this induces Faraday's Law of Induction (physics again). This process induces microcurrents in every cell in the body. The PEMF is literally recharging the cells, or to put it another way, it's increasing the cellular voltage potential. This is the same physics that is used in a generator to generate currents or in a pad charger to charge your smart phone's battery.

'Electricity puts into the tired body just what it needs most... life force, nerve force. It's a great doctor, I can tell you, perhaps the greatest of all doctors.' – Nikola Tesla

On one level, cells work like a battery. All cells have a voltage and that voltage governs much of the efficiency of the biochemistry and metabolism in the body. If individuals have a low cellular voltage, just like a low battery, the body isn't as efficient as it could be in communicating, signaling, repairing and maintaining a state of health. Therefore, if the body increases cellular voltage, it increases metabolic, biochemical and bioelectrical efficiencies. In turn it improves or enhances the body's potential to do what it needs to do to restore or preserve a healthy balance or homeostasis.

Another reason we need to charge the cells is because low voltage is linked with many chronic disorders and with any injury that is slow to heal. For example, it is known that damaged or diseased cells often present an abnormally low voltage potential, which can be up to 80% lower than healthy cells. There may be other imbalances, deficiencies or toxins contributing to the problem. There may be also improper nutrition, bad lifestyle, stress, emotions and negative environmental and social impacts.

PEMF therapy addresses a fundamental bioelectric deficiency in the cells. One way you can look at PEMF therapy is to call it voltage or energy supplementation. This is why PEMF works for so many disorders... because one of the associated properties of many of those disorders is a low cellular voltage potential. It is just common sense and is not addressed by Western medicine. Conventional Western medicine does not address the biophysics or the bioelectric nature of the body. They measure and use the data for analysis from electrocardiograms (ECG or EKG), electroencephalograms (EEG) and electromyograms (EMG), which measure biopotentials or the electrical output of the heart, brain and muscles.

Frequently Asked Questions about PEMF

Can I use PEMF, if I have a metal implants (surgical screws, staples, plates)?

Yes, you can use low intensity PEMF therapy if you have any sort of metal implants, surgical screws, staples, plates, stents, knee, shoulder or hip replacements made of any material with a low intensity system. I highly suggest you check with the manufacturer of any high intensity system about using their product with any metal implants within the body. However, as mentioned early in the book, you can't use PEMF to treat people who have epilepsy, battery operated implanted devices, are pregnant or have an organ transplant.

Does it matter if I eat before or after a treatment?

No, it doesn't make any difference when you eat at all. It's best to drink some water before and right after a PEMF treatment. The more hydrated you are, the longer you hold the cellular charge from the treatment and PEMF can be a little dehydrating, especially if the far infrared is also activated on the mat.

The benefits of far infrared with PEMF

Far infrared therapy uses far infrared light, a segment of the spectrum of sunlight. Unlike ultraviolet light, which can damage the skin, far infrared light is safe and beneficial. It penetrates the skin reaching muscles, tissues and organs, which promotes various health benefits.

Key Benefits

1. Pain Relief and Management

- **Reduces Chronic Pain:** FIR therapy is effective in alleviating chronic pain conditions such as arthritis, fibromyalgia and lower back pain by improving blood circulation and reducing inflammation.

- **Eases Muscle and Joint Pain:** Athletes and active individuals benefit from reduced muscle soreness and faster recovery times, thanks to FIR's ability to relax muscles and joints.

2. Improved Circulation

- **Enhances Blood Flow:** FIR therapy promotes vasodilation, which increases blood flow and oxygen delivery to tissues, enhancing overall cardiovascular health.

- **Supports Detoxification:** Improved circulation aids in the removal of toxins and waste products from the body, promoting better detoxification.

3. Enhanced Skin Health

- **Rejuvenates Skin:** FIR therapy boosts collagen production, improving skin elasticity and reducing the appearance of wrinkles and fine lines.

- **Treats Skin Conditions:** Conditions such as eczema, psoriasis and acne can benefit from the anti-inflammatory and healing properties of FIR.

4. Boosted Immune Function

- **Strengthens Immunity:** Regular FIR therapy sessions can enhance the immune system by promoting better circulation and detoxification, leading to increased resilience against illnesses.

- **Reduces Inflammation:** The anti-inflammatory effects of FIR can help manage autoimmune conditions and support overall immune health.

5. Stress Relief and Relaxation

- **Promotes Relaxation:** FIR therapy induces deep relaxation by soothing the nervous system, reducing stress, and promoting a sense of well-being.

- **Improves Sleep:** Many users report improved sleep quality after FIR sessions, as the therapy aids in reducing anxiety and promoting relaxation.

6. Weight Loss and Metabolism Boost

- **Aids Weight Loss:** FIR therapy can increase metabolism and promote calorie burning, assisting in weight loss efforts.

- **Reduces Cellulite:** By improving circulation and skin health, FIR can also help reduce the appearance of cellulite.

Is it safe to use on children or older adults?

Since this is a low intensity system that generates natural electromagnetic waves right around or below the earth's natural magnetic field intensity, then this is safe to treat children and adults of all ages. It's best not to treat infants less than one month old just to play it safe. I would never use a high intensity system on a young developing child.

Can PEMF therapy help me or a loved one?

One of the first questions people ask is if PEMF can help them. I always say that I don't really know, because, I don't. I can only tell how it has helped other people with a similar problem in the past. I can't answer for everyone specifically, because as I've said before, everyone is different.

There are many variables in play with each individual regarding their lifestyle, emotions and mental outlook, which all have an influence. All I can tell them is to have some treatments.

Wounds don't heal overnight, so neither does anything else if it is truly healing. Masking agents can work quickly for pain, but we all know there can be consequences with long term use of drugs. Yes, I've seen pain subside significantly with one PEMF treatment, but that's an exception to the rule. High intensity PEMF systems are used effectively to reduce pain quickly, especially for professional sports. On the other hand, some biophysicists and medical professionals believe that high intensity PEMF systems numb the neural pain receptors, which is the same thing as masking the pain.

As a general rule-of-thumb, PEMF helps about 80% of the people I see. I scratch my head in wonder when it doesn't help someone who has a similar problem to other people where it did help. Therein lies the differences within people again. There are just too many variables in people's lives, their bodies, hearts and minds that may have a significant impact on the success or failure of PEMF to be a benefit for everyone.

CHAPTER 5
PEMF Systems & Devices

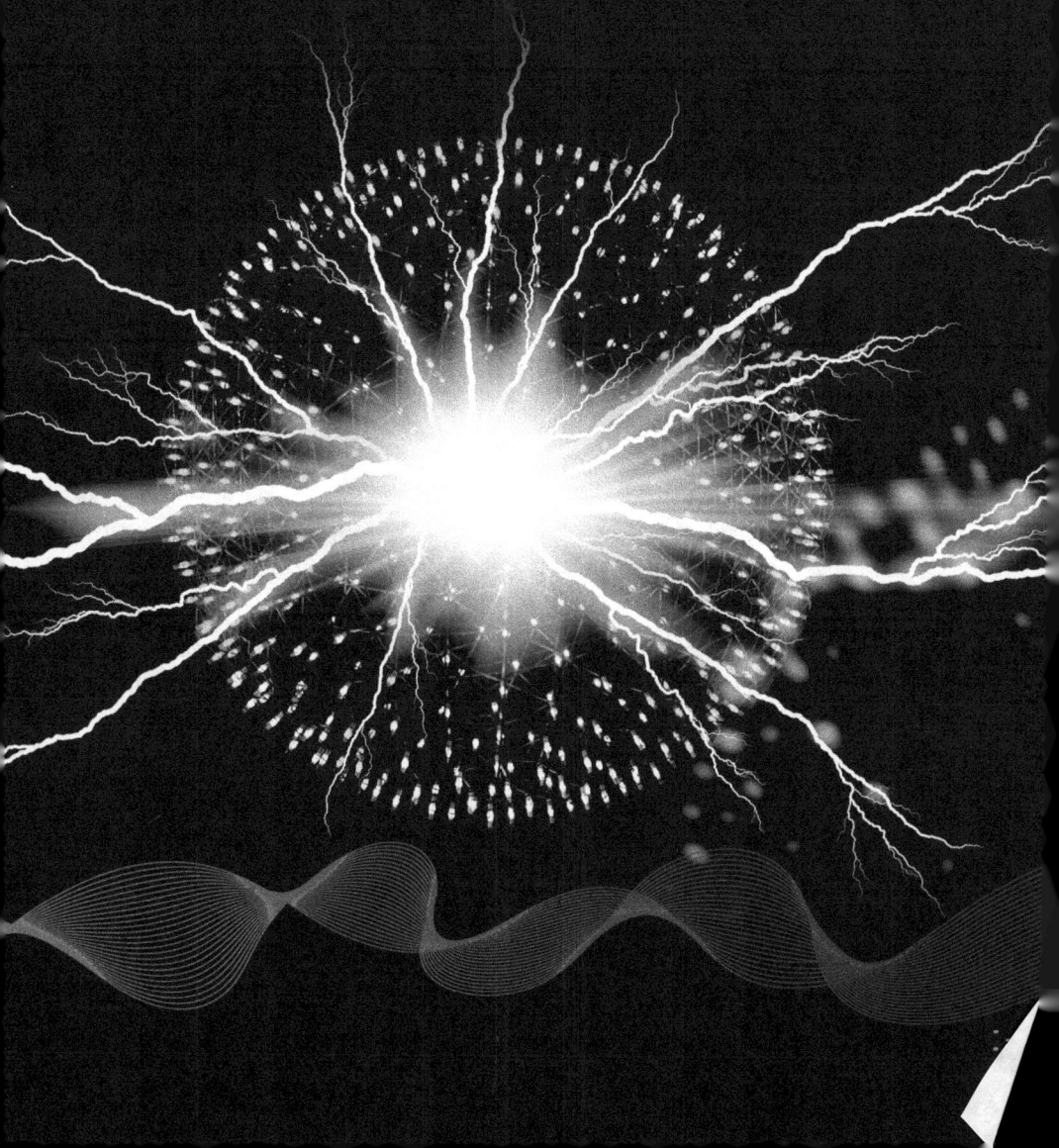

CHAPTER 5

PEMF Systems & Devices

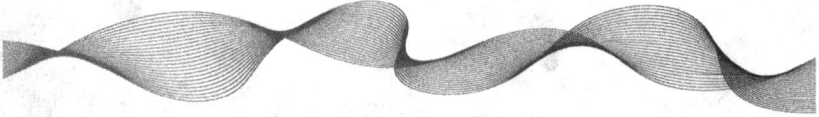

Types of PEMF Devices

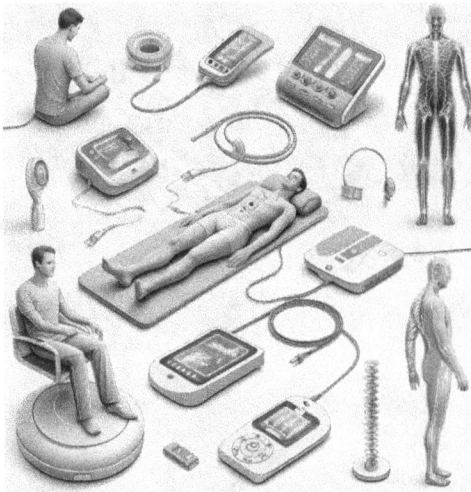

PEMF therapy has seen a significant rise in popularity in recent years due to its numerous health benefits, which range from pain relief to improved sleep and enhanced tissue repair. As the demand has grown, a variety of systems have emerged on the market to cater to different needs, preferences and budgets. As a result, it's very confusing with experts of varying degrees saying you must use a certain intensity, frequency or type of PEMF system.

The market has also been flooded with cheap counterfeit or fake PEMF systems that do little or nothing much at all. Along with this there are other techno gadgets that purport to do marvelous things touting words like quantum energy, frequency, optical crystal/ quartz, Tesla, photonic, vibration, auric, ionic, virtual and so on. Be careful and do your research.

In this chapter, I will explain the types of PEMF devices available for the general public, along with their advantages and disadvantages in regard to the different kinds of hardware configurations and applicators that emit the PEMFs. I will delve much deeper into the high versus low intensity debate in Chapter 7, which is very confusing to many people and needs far more explanation.

1. Full-body Mat Systems:

- **Description**: Full-body mat systems consist of a large mat embedded with multiple copper coils along with additional localized applicators. The mats are similar in size to a yoga mat. Users lie on the mat and receive PEMF therapy through every cell in the body. Their localized applicators are used to focus the PEMF on specific areas of the body.

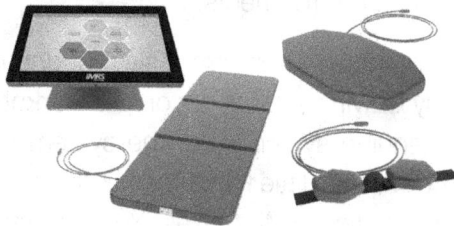

PEMF System with 3 Applicators

- **Advantages**: A full-body mat system is my first priority over any other PEMF system.

  - Comprehensive coverage: These mats provide PEMFs to the entire body simultaneously, making them convenient for overall wellness. Also, as stated before, where a problem manifests in the body may not necessarily be the single source of the problem. It's common to get referral pains where the location of the pain is not the same as the source of the problem. Sciatic pain (sciatica) that runs down the back of the leg can originate from the lower back. Full-body mats literally cover all the bases.

- Localized applicators: Many whole-body systems offer additional and smaller targeted PEMF applicators along with the whole-body mat for more localized treatments.

- Ease of use: Users simply lie on the mat to receive therapy, making it suitable for passive use during activities like reading, watching TV or meditating.

- **Disadvantages:**

  - Cost: Full-body mat systems tend to be more expensive compared to other types of PEMF devices.

  - Portability: Due to their size, these mats may not be easily portable, limiting their use to home or health practice environments.

  - Counterfeits: There are a slew of cheap or fake whole-body PEMF systems out on the market. They are copies of genuine systems like the system I use. They either produce very little PEMF or flux density or don't produce therapeutic PEMFs at all. You can still read wonderful testimonial about them, but anyone can say anything on the internet.

2. Portable Devices:

- **Description**: Portable PEMF devices are smaller, handheld devices that deliver targeted PEMF therapy to specific areas of the body.

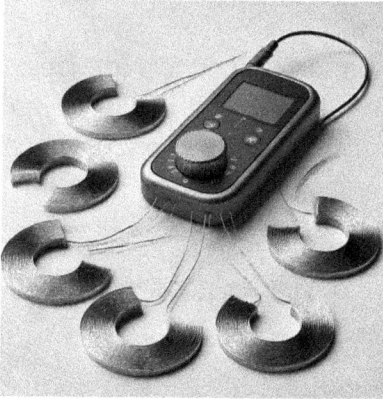

- **Advantages**:

- Targeted therapy: Users can direct PEMF therapy to specific areas of pain or discomfort, allowing for more precise treatment.

- Portability: These devices are lightweight and compact, making them suitable for travel or use on-the-go.

- **Disadvantages**:

  - Limited coverage: Portable devices may only provide therapy to a small area at a time, requiring multiple sessions for treating all of the body.

  - Power constraints: Portable devices may have limited power and battery life compared to larger systems, potentially affecting the intensity or effectiveness of therapy.

3. **Pad Systems:**

- **Description**: pad systems consist of various sized pads embedded with PEMF coils. Users can lay or wrap the pads around specific body parts to target localized areas.

- **Advantages**:

  - Flexibility: pad systems allow users to target specific areas of the body with ease, making them versatile for addressing various types of pain or injury.

  - Moderate cost: pad systems typically cost less than full-body mat systems while still providing targeted therapy.

- **Disadvantages**:

  - Limited coverage: Similar to portable devices, pad systems may only provide therapy to a small area at a time. This requires multiple treatments on different areas of the body.

  - Comfort: Depending on the design, some users may find it uncomfortable to wear or position the pads for extended periods.

4. Chair or Seat Cushion Devices:

- **Description**: These devices are integrated into chairs or seat cushions, allowing users to receive PEMF therapy while seated.

- **Advantages**:

  - Convenience: Users can receive PEMF therapy while performing other tasks, such as working at a desk.

  - Targeted therapy: These devices often target the lower back and buttocks area, which are common areas of tension and discomfort.

- **Disadvantages**:

  - Limited coverage: Chair or seat cushion devices only provide therapy to specific areas of the body, excluding other regions that may benefit from treatment.

5. Wearable Devices:

- **Description**: Wearable PEMF devices are worn directly on the body, such as bracelets, wraps or belts, delivering localized therapy throughout the day.

Advantages:

- Continuous therapy: Wearable devices provide continuous PEMF therapy while allowing users to remain active and mobile.

- Discreetness: Some of these devices can be worn discreetly under clothing, allowing users to receive therapy without drawing attention.

Disadvantages:

- Limited power: Wearable devices may have limited power compared to larger systems, potentially affecting the intensity or effectiveness of therapy. There's also the issue of batteries or battery charging.

- Limited coverage: Due to their compact size, wearable devices can only provide therapy to a very small area of the body at a time.

In conclusion, the variety of PEMF devices available on the market provide users options to tailor their therapy to their specific needs and preferences. Whether seeking comprehensive full-body treatment or targeted relief for specific areas, individuals can choose from a range of devices that suit their lifestyle and budget. However, it's essential to consider the advantages and disadvantages of each type before making a decision to ensure the most effective and suitable therapy for individual wellness goals.

CHAPTER 6
Detoxification

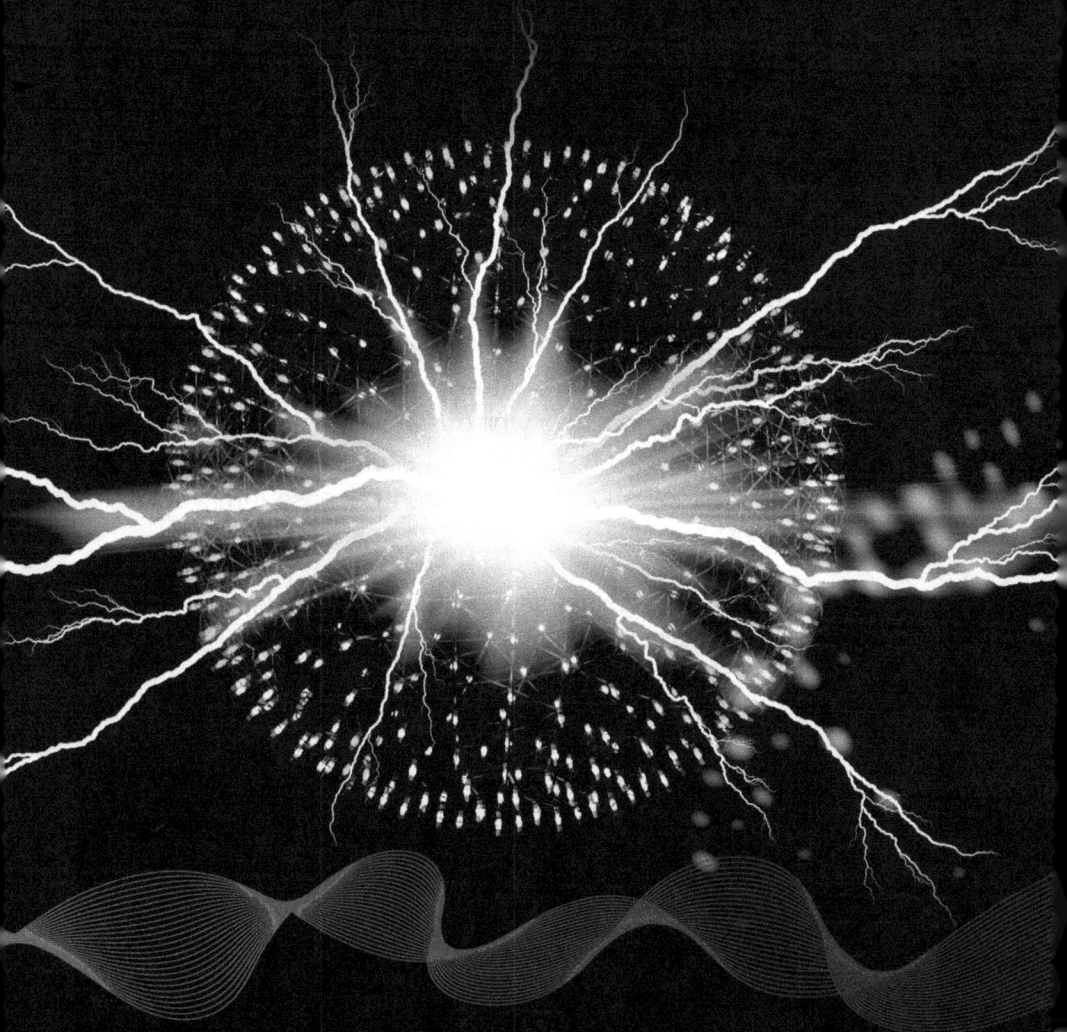

CHAPTER 6

Detoxification

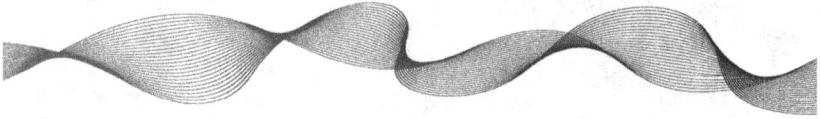

Detoxification is the neutralization and elimination of toxins and natural metabolic wastes from the body. Detoxification is good for you. It shows that your body is positively responding to a therapy or treatment of some kind, even if it's unpleasant at first. Two steps back before going forward with some favorable results.

When researching PEMF on the internet, you don't hear much about any side effects of PEMF, especially with high intensity systems. Many manufacturers say there are no side effects while others simply don't mention anything at all. Most websites list the contraindications, which are specific situations or conditions in which PEMF therapy should not be used because it may have deleterious effects.

PEMF therapy does have a side effect. The side effect is detoxification along with a little dehydration. Detoxification is a good sign that the body is beginning to respond to the therapy, but it needs to be done slowly. Detoxification can be experienced in many different ways. On some level, whether a person is aware of it or not, detoxification will be a part of the process. The good thing is that over 50% of people will not notice anything at all if they slowly and gradually get accustomed to the PEMFs, especially in regard to intensity.

The process of detoxification and elimination

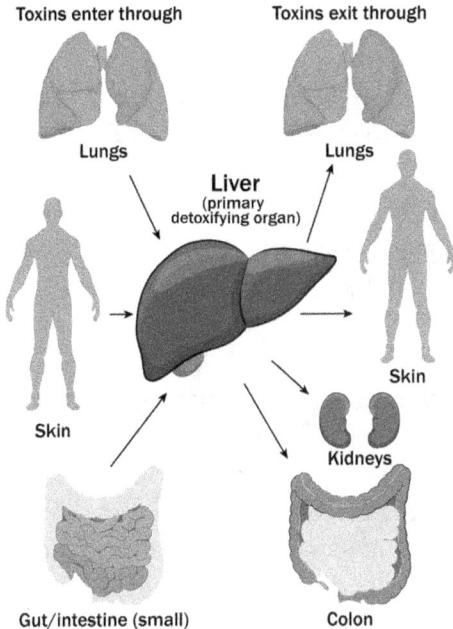

Toxins enter through

Toxins exit through

Lungs

Lungs

Liver
(primary
detoxifying organ)

Skin

Skin

Kidneys

Gut/intestine (small)

Colon

It can take some time for the body to acclimate to PEMF, which will vary with everyone. The rule of thumb is several days for the organs of elimination (liver, kidneys, lungs, colon and skin) to catch up by increasing their metabolic efficiency to handle the increase release of wastes that PEMF can stimulate. What you don't want to happen is for the cells to start releasing metabolic wastes and potential toxins too fast. If you follow the time and intensity treatment protocols, 95% of the time you're not going to have any problems with detoxification where the experience is disruptive and pain or symptoms are significantly amplified. Always start using a low intensity and the recommended amount of time. This is especially important when using a whole-body mat.

Detoxification prevents metabolic waste products from accumulating in the body and impeding natural functions, which can affect the overall state of your health. Some people may experience a PEMF detox to some degree after their first treatment or subsequent treatments. It doesn't happen with everyone, but it's not uncommon either. PEMF enhances the efficiency of your physiology and biochemistry at the cellular level. Again, detoxification is a good sign that PEMF is working and that the body is responding positively.

We just want the response to be a gradual increase in efficiency, so the body can effectively eliminate all of the metabolic wastes and potential toxins, if present.

The topic of toxins normally comes up in discussions about detoxification. If the body is detoxifying, then it's also going to be eliminating toxins, *if present*. Toxins and metabolic wastes are generally woven together. On one level, a metabolic waste is a toxin. Everyone that experiences PEMF therapy is going to have some degree of detoxification whether they feel it or not, even if it's just a slight dehydration of the body.

It's very difficult to tell if the detox is coming from increased metabolic wastes, toxins or both. The good thing is that most of the time, it's usually just a minor issue with little or no symptoms. To diminish the potential of negative effects, always drink at least one glass of water before a PEMF treatment and immediately after a treatment. You do this for two reasons: 1 – the more hydrated you are, the longer you hold the cellular charge you're receiving from the treatment.

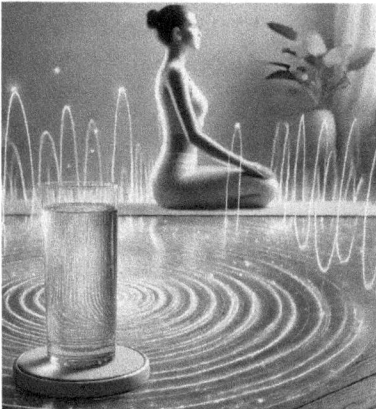

2 – water helps to clear out any potential increase in metabolic wastes or toxins. It's highly recommended to drink six to eight glasses of water per day.

If the detoxification is a bit too disruptive, which it rarely is, then it's advisable to enlist the support of a healthcare provider who is experienced with detoxification. Many of the people I see have already enlisted the aid of a health provider like a nutritionist or naturopath to take a more holistic and proactive approach. Some kind of binder may be necessary to enhance the capture and elimination of the toxins using activated charcoal, apple pectin, chlorophyll or clays (bentonite/zeolite). There are many different kinds of binders that bond with the toxins, which facilitates their elimination. Again, it's a rare happening in my experience, but it is a good idea to talk to a health professional that is trained to deal with the elimination of toxins.

Detoxing individuals who are reacting to the release of toxins may also experience an accelerated depletion of nutrients, which can necessitate the need for additional supplementation. Again, seeking the guidance from a professional nutritional consult may be advisable. As an aside, the increase in cellular efficiency from PEMF will automatically increase the rate of absorption of nutrients and elimination, therefore it is a very good adjunct for nutritionists or naturopaths to add to their practice along with many other kinds of complementary health practices.

"PEMF is the ultimate adjunct therapy. PEMF works well with all forms of therapy because it reduces chronic pathological inflammatory states within the body. This in turn improves the effects and efficiency of many other therapies." – Dr Robert Dennis - Prof of Biomedical Engineering at the University of North Carolina.

In essence, PEMF increases cellular charge or the voltage potential of the cells. This increased charge, just like charging a battery, makes the cells metabolically more efficient or active. Therefore, the most common kind of detoxification is going to be an increase in metabolic wastes coming out of the cells. Toxins may be also present.

As an example, let's say your body is running at an energy level of 5 as your personal benchmark. This is your normal baseline cellular efficiency and everything is hopefully functioning smoothly. Through the introduction of PEMF therapy, we increase cellular efficiency by 10% to 15% over the whole body. Suddenly, metabolic wastes that have been systematically eliminated at the regular rate of 5, get eliminated 10% to 15% quicker. Your body, especially the organs of elimination, hasn't had enough time to adjust to the newly acquired metabolic efficiency needed to manage the increased waste production from the cells. There is usually a time lag for the organs of elimination to catch up and be able to deal with the increased release of metabolic wastes. Sometimes this can take a couple of days. Most of the time it's a non-issue if you err on the side of caution and go easy with the intensity. Just use the standard initial treatment protocols for PEMF treatments using a whole-body mat.

In my experience, most people don't notice much of anything in regard to any detoxification. Some may notice a kind of sluggishness or low energy for a period of time… possibly a headache. The period of time can vary from hours to a few days, but usually not much longer. I've had people report that they felt like they may be coming down with something… like you sometimes feel before getting ill. Others have reported an increase in brain fog, headaches or even an increased pain in a problem area. Other symptom of detoxification can be dizziness, skin eruptions, diarrhea and sleep disruptions. As I said, I don't find this to be a major problem because I always start people off on a set time with a low intensity to reduce the potential so the body can acclimate.

Also, if everyone knows about the potential for detoxification, then this will make life far less stressful. When some degree of reaction to PEMF happens, I always say that it's a good sign that PEMF is beginning to work. This may not be what people want to hear. But, when you clean house, you're bound to raise a bit of dust. My other analogy: when you drain the swamp, there's going to be some muck that needs to be cleared out. People who have some level of a healing reaction, sometimes called a Herxheimer reaction, have a higher probability that they will begin to see benefits or reduction of their symptoms sooner than someone who doesn't react at all. This is if they continue with the treatments and don't stop. How long it takes to go through a detox is very individual, but it's usually one to three days for the vast majority of people.

There are six ways to eliminate wastes or toxins. This is through the skin, the lungs (CO_2), kidneys, liver, colon and lymphatic system. The liver plays the biggest part in this process and PEMF therapy has the capability to improve the functions of inefficient livers and also the kidneys. Both organs are extremely important in the process of elimination or detoxification. PEMF helps to optimize the organ's ability to function in a more effective manner, thus helping the body with its natural detoxification process.

There is one question I like to ask everyone before I start a treatment and that is if they consider themselves to be sensitive. Almost everyone that is 'sensitive' already knows it. If they say yes, then I'll turn the intensity down below the standard protocol. If there is hesitation to my question, then I figure they aren't sensitive, but you can always err on the side of caution.

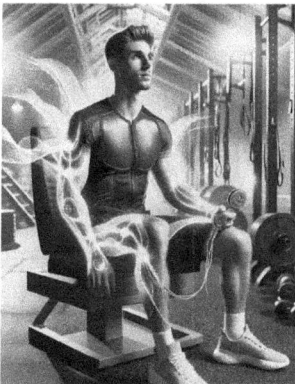

Athletes have a tendency to respond the quickest and very favorably to PEMF. They are also notorious for being gung-ho. I rented a PEMF system to a serious runner one time in the distant past. With my rental system, you set two parameters on the control unit: time in minutes and intensity at specific levels within the control unit. People usually start out at ten or fifteen minutes at an intensity of 25 or 50, which is on the lower scale setting of intensity. This is what I recommend.

Almost everyone thinks 'more is better' and such was the case of a gung-ho athlete who rented the system. He decided on his own, which was counter to the instructions, to go sixty minutes at an intensity of 400. This is the highest possible setting for both minutes and intensity on the system. Several hours later after vomiting and diarrhea, he called me to report the detox reaction. What was so surprising to him was that he didn't feel anything during the time on the whole-body mat. I hope it's clear that you don't have to 'feel' anything for PEMF therapy to be working.

I have to tell one more story about my experience with detoxification, which was early on in my practice. I had a guy contact me who wanted to bring over his super-duper PEMF mat to show me. He had one of those systems that purports to produce PEMF along with far infrared, negative ions, red light therapy and healing crystals. I was curious and wanted to see one of these 'special' systems that lures a certain segment of the market with all its bells and whistles along with a very cheap price.

He brought the mat over to my clinic. I didn't try his mat but gave him a go on my whole-body mat. He said he'd been doing PEMF for over nine months, so I figured his body had acclimated to PEMF over that amount of time. No need to worry about any detox for him! So, I turned the mat up to 200 for only ten minutes. Relatively speaking when compared to high intensity systems, this is still a very, very low intensity. A high-intensity guru would say it doesn't even go through the whole body, but my TriField electromagnetic field meter proves this to be wrong. I get plenty of signal strength going all the way through the body and several feet above it.

I got a call two or three days after the treatment and the gentleman had been very sick with flu-like symptoms for at last two days. He couldn't go to work and still sounded pretty low in energy. He had a major detoxification. I really felt bad. So, the lesson for me was not to assume acclimation to PEMF from these cheap systems that say they can do everything. Some of these systems have been shown to produce no resonating PEMFs at all. I can only assume that he detoxed because his system wasn't producing much or any PEMF at all.

What does detoxification look like

Detoxification is good for the body, but the process can initially produce some symptoms. Some of the most common are:

- Fatigue or sluggishness
- Increased pain or inflammation in problem areas
- Metallic taste in the mouth (possibly a sign of heavy metals)
- Sleep disruption
- Skin rash or redness
- Nausea
- Diarrhea
- Anxiety
- Shortness of breath
- Brain fog
- Slight fever
- Headaches, dizziness
- Foul breath and/or body odor
- Itching
- Tingling feeling

What's interesting about the list above is that the opposite reactions become some of the most common benefits people see from PEMF therapy. This is why I like to see some kind of mild side effect, because I know that PEMF is beginning to work. Hopefully it's simply a matter of taking a couple of steps backwards before going positively forward.

In dealing with the treatment of any chronic or acute condition, a detoxification or healing reaction can arise in approximately 10% to 15% of the people treated in the first few days or week. This can manifest as an increase in the symptoms associated with the problem, like pain for example. It can sometimes cause an aggravation, or what people might call, a stirring or shifting inside of them. This may enhance the problem or in some way focus more of their attention on it, but hopefully not in an uncomfortable manner. Detoxification may also be expected at some level after a prolonged period of medication. So, it's best to be gentle in regards to time and intensity with a PEMF treatment. Just know that everyone will detox to some degree, it's just that most won't know it if you take it slow and easy by using a low intensity.

Some people may experience a light itching on some parts of the body or a warm tingling feeling may be felt. In exactly the same manner, bruises, cramps, strains, wounds or issues with the joints and back may make themselves known as light tingling or pain as a result of the increase of the circulation. If previously unnoticed physical reactions become noticeable along with the application of PEMF therapy, then consultation with an experienced therapist in PEMF is recommended. Again, for me it's all a very good sign that the body is responding. As a general rule, those who do show some sign of detoxification have a higher probability of seeing a good result if they stick with the therapy and work through it. It usually doesn't take very long. Most of the time it's one of two days, if it happens at all.

Managing detoxification

The first course of action if there is some level of detoxification is to drink lots of water. Most people don't drink nearly enough water. In fact, it's estimated that 90% of the general population is dehydrated on some level. I recommend eight glasses of water per day as a normal routine. Experienced health professionals say that dehydration is one of the most common or contributing factors to many kinds of disorders. Always drink lots of good water and I mean just water, not tea, coffee or carbonated drinks with sugar… just clean and pure water of the best quality you can get.

Another course of action for detoxification is to immediately reduce the number of treatments, reduce the magnetic field intensity or stop altogether. This allows the body to clear itself of toxins or wastes while also acclimating to the increase in cellular efficiency. This should be done for as long as it takes for the symptoms to settle back down. That amount of time will vary for everyone. There needs to be a good level of communication with the appropriate person to determine the best course of action. Some people like to push or bull their way through the detoxification on one end of the scale, while others can become afraid or concerned and just want it to go away or even stop the treatments. It's sad sometimes to lose someone who reacts strongly to PEMF because that reaction is a good sign that things are actually going in the right direction, even though it appears to be the opposite at the moment.

CHAPTER 7

Intensity: High vs Low-Intensity PEMF Systems

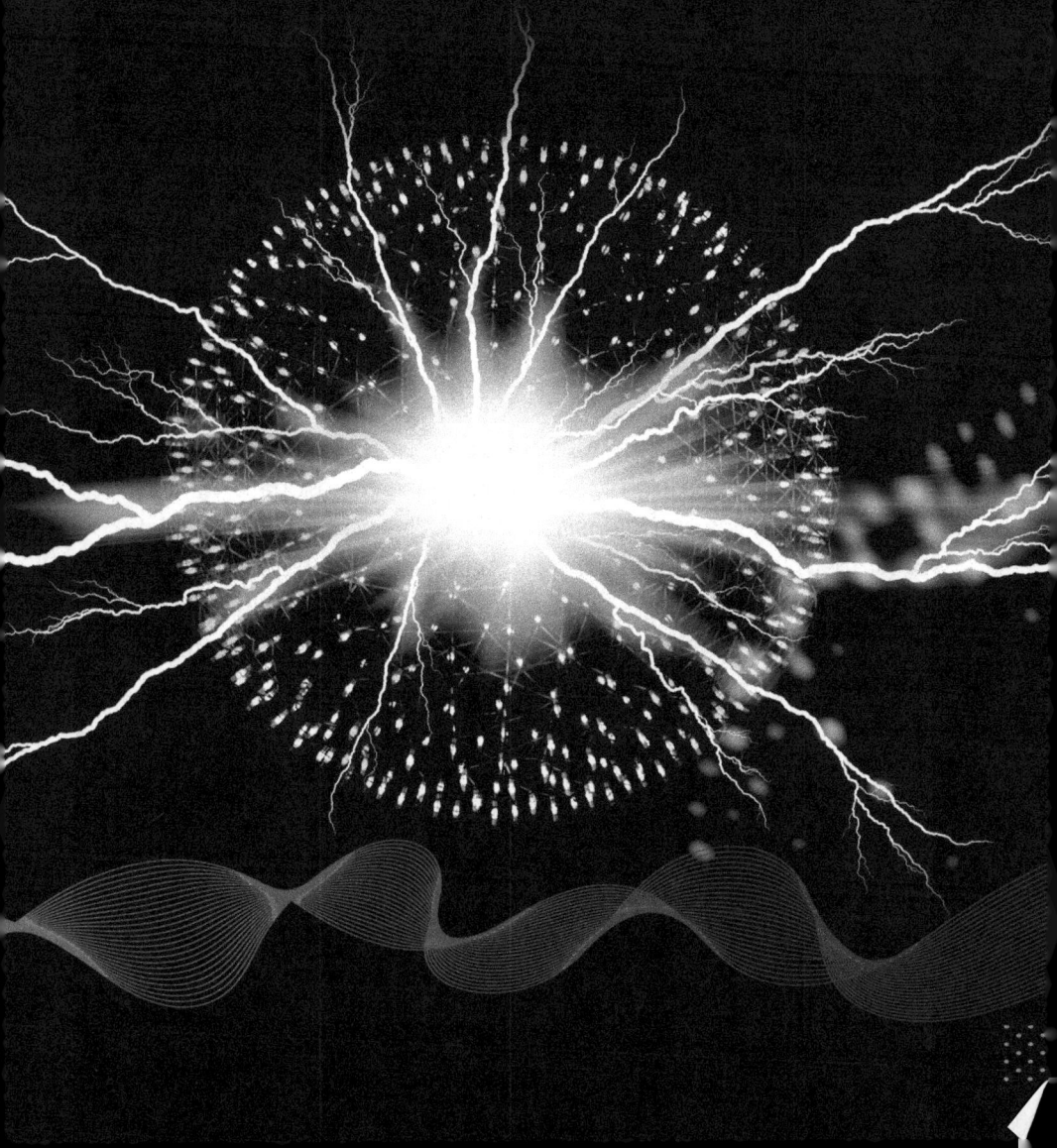

CHAPTER 7

Intensity: High vs Low-Intensity PEMF Systems

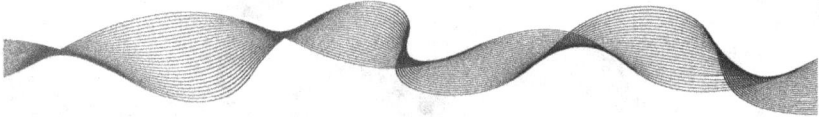

There is a *lot* of debate about intensity or the amplitude/strength of electromagnetic fields in the PEMF world, especially if you are looking at purchasing a system. People find it very confusing due to the two prevailing schools of thought about intensity. There is the *'more is better'* school advocating high intensity and then there's what I call the natural or earth-based approach using low intensity - *'less is more.'*

I am openly biased toward low intensity and also low frequency systems. I use them in my clinic, I also rent and sell low intensity systems. To me, it's simply common sense to resonate with the natural frequencies *and intensities* of the cells and not over modulate or hit them with an astounding big hammer using high intensities. Harmony, resonance and coherence versus over stimulation, over modulation or cellular dissonance. So, if you are of the high intensity persuasion, then the following chapter is probably not going to *resonate* with you.

"Clinical and behavioral research validates the 'less is more' principle of energetic interactions. Convincing evidence came in 1975, when a number of scientists confirmed that extremely weak (low intensity), low frequency electric fields can have significant effects on important regulatory processes in the brain. These findings led to the concept of the power/ frequency window, which is a narrow range of signal properties that will produce a maximum biological effect." – Dr James L. Oschman – 'Energy and the Healing Response' and author of Energy Medicine.

My Opinion on High Intensity vs Low Intensity

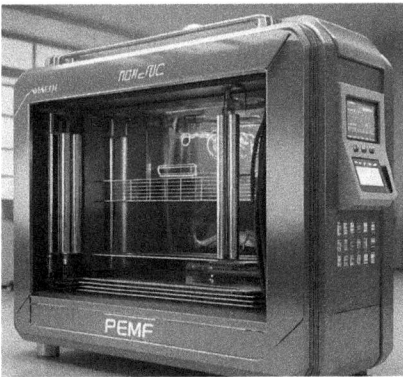

I'm not going to spend too much time discussing high intensity PEMF systems or their use. There is a place for them to attend to acute pain, severe bone fractures, drug-resistant depression, but only in a clinical setting and administered by a licensed healthcare professional.

Unfortunately, this is not the case. As noted previously, there is currently little or no regulation on the use of PEMF machines in most countries at this time. The strength of the electromagnetic fields that high intensity systems generate can approach the levels of an MRI (magnetic resonance imaging) scanner. This is *way* outside the Safe Zone set by the International Commission on Non-ionizing Radiation Protection (ICNIRP). That's enough for me to read the signs of common sense and err on the side of caution, especially if using it on people.

I've purchased five other types of systems and the one I currently use I feel is the safest and most full featured PEMF system on the market. I've taken several PEMF training courses by one doctor in the US who is regarded as an authority on PEMF. He repeatedly says in his courses that high intensity systems should only be used by a licensed and trained healthcare professional. The reality is that he sells high intensity PEMF systems to *anyone* on his website.

Here are some general distinctions between high-intensity and low-intensity PEMF devices:

1. Field Strength:

- **Low-Intensity PEMF Devices:** These devices have field strengths ranging from 0.5 microtesla (μT) to around 1000 microtesla (μT) or 10 gauss. They are considered to have milder effects due to use of more natural or earth-based electromagnetic fields in regard to both intensity and frequency. The earth produces electromagnetic waves that we have lived and evolved within over eons. Low intensity PEMF systems produced similar electromagnetic waves in line with the earth.

- **High-Intensity PEMF Devices:** Can have field strengths ranging from 10 millitesla (mT) to several Tesla (T). 1 Tesla equals 10,000 gauss. This would be around 20,000 times stronger than the earth's natural magnetic field strength. Some high intensity PEMF systems go even higher.

2. Treatment Duration:

- **Low-Intensity PEMF Devices:** Often used for longer durations with the treatment sessions lasting from fifteen minutes up to an hour or more.

- **High-Intensity PEMF Devices:** Treatment sessions with high-intensity devices are typically shorter, often ranging from a few minutes to around 30 minutes.

3. Application and Purpose:

- **Low-Intensity PEMF Devices:** Commonly used for many different kinds of health conditions, general well-being, relaxation, rejuvenation and to support overall health and maintenance. They may be used as part of daily routines for existing chronic conditions or preventive and supportive care.

- **High-Intensity PEMF Devices:** These devices are often used for more acute therapeutic applications on people. At present, the majority of use of these systems is on horses. The last market share report I read stated that 73% of high intensity systems are used on horses. With people, this type of system should only be used under the supervision of a licensed health professional.

- To repeat, there no regulations on the use of PEMF devices at this time, so my advice is to be very careful with whom you choose for a PEMF treatment, especially with high intensity systems. Be sure to ask what type of system they use. If they hesitate or are unsure with their answer, then this may be a sign that they don't have much experience.

4. Professional vs. Home Use:

- **Low-Intensity PEMF Devices:** Many low-intensity devices are designed for home and professional use, depending on the system. They are very user-friendly and more suitable for daily professional or self-administration use.

- **High-Intensity PEMF Devices:** Most high-intensity devices are intended for use in professional healthcare settings under the guidance of trained and licensed healthcare practitioner. They require more specialized knowledge for safe and effective application and are generally used to treat acute cases.

It's important to note that the appropriateness of a PEMF device may depend on individual health conditions. Consulting with an experienced healthcare professional who is also trained in PEMF is advisable before seeking PEMF therapy, especially for specific therapeutic purposes. The Catch-22 is that many healthcare providers don't know much or anything about PEMF at this time. Additionally, the specific waveform, frequency and other parameters of the PEMF signal and construction of the PEMF device can also influence its effects. Some of the cheap systems don't produce any *therapeutic PEMF waves* at all. These factors should also be considered along with intensity when evaluating PEMF devices. For the layman, it can get very complicated

With respect to high intensity systems, I've heard and read some good things about high intensity PEMF, but I've also heard some negative stories. The negative stories I hear usually come from people who have gone to see someone for a high intensity treatment who has graduated from treating horses to people. Most of these people are involved in or related to the world of horses in some manner. They are not like my integrative doctor who has a

Swiss manufactured high intensity system that he says is good for quick pain reduction and other acute traumas. I personally have not used his system and prefer to completely stay away from all high intensity systems based on common sense, intuition and some of the research I'll get to later on.

Again, and this is just my opinion. High intensity systems may have their place in clinical settings for the moment. I do believe that high intensity should never be used daily or on any kind of regular or repeated basis. In my opinion, along with several experts in the field, and also according to the ICNIRP (International Commission on Non-Ionizing Radiation Protection) high intensity systems are dangerous.

On the other hand, a low-intensity PEMF system is a very suitable and safe choice for daily use if it's below 5 gauss. Here are some things to consider:

1. **Safety:** Low-intensity PEMF systems are considered safe for home or professional use. High-intensity systems should only be used by a licensed healthcare professional. Note: see *Safety of PEMF* at the end of this chapter.

2. **Versatility:** Low-intensity PEMF systems are often more versatile and can be used for a variety of applications, including pain relief, sleep improvement, depression/anxiety and overall wellness.

3. **Cost:** Low-intensity systems are usually more affordable than high-intensity systems, making them a more cost-effective option for individuals on a budget.

4. **Ease of Use:** Low-intensity PEMF devices are often designed for easy and convenient use.

5. **Portability**: Many low-intensity PEMF devices are light, compact and portable, allowing their use in different locations.

6. **Effects**: High-intensity PEMF systems may lead to stronger and more immediate effects, which might not be suitable for everyone. Low-intensity systems provide a milder approach that is generally well-tolerated.

7. **Wellness Maintenance**: Low-intensity PEMF systems can be suitable for general wellness maintenance and preventive care, providing gentle support for overall health.

8. **Risk of Side Effects**: High-intensity PEMF systems may have a higher risk of side effects such as skin irritation or discomfort. Low-intensity systems are designed to minimize such risks.

9. **Duration of Use**: Low-intensity PEMF sessions can often be used for longer durations without causing discomfort, allowing users to incorporate them into their daily routines more easily.

10. **Accessibility**: Low-intensity PEMF systems are more accessible to a broader range of individuals, including those with specific health conditions or sensitivities that may preclude the use of higher intensity devices.

11. **Health Conditions**: Low-intensity PEMF systems may be more suitable for individuals with chronic conditions or those seeking long-term, ongoing use. High-intensity systems may be more targeted for specific or acute therapeutic interventions.

12. **Non-Invasiveness**: Low-intensity PEMF systems are generally non-invasive and present a lower risk of causing discomfort or harm from muscle contractions. This makes them a preferable

option for individuals who are sensitive to intense treatments. This is one of the reasons most clinical research that's done on PEMF is low intensity.

13. **Integration with Other Therapies:** Low-intensity PEMF systems can be easily integrated into existing wellness routines and may complement other therapeutic approaches. They are often used alongside conventional medical treatments for a holistic approach to health.

14. **Research and Evidence**: There is far more research done and therefore more evidence and clinical studies supporting the use of low-intensity PEMF for many different kinds of health conditions, as opposed to high-intensity systems.

15. **Maintenance**: Low-intensity PEMF systems often require little or no maintenance and have fewer components that can wear out or malfunction over time compared to high-intensity systems. My system requires periodic firmware updates only. Spark gap high intensity systems require expensive periodic maintenance depending on the amount of use.

16. **Preventive Health**: Low-intensity PEMF systems may be more aligned with preventive health measures, promoting overall wellness and potentially reducing the risk of certain health issues.

17. **Individual Sensitivity**: Individuals vary in their sensitivity to electromagnetic fields. Some may find low-intensity PEMF systems more comfortable, especially if they are new to PEMF therapy, while others may be able to tolerate higher intensities as well.

I want to apologize for this next section if it gets a bit technical, but it's important to address the confusion about high versus low intensity.

Understanding Intensity

'*Buy the highest intensity PEMF machine that you can afford… you can always turn it down.*' – These are the actual words written by a PEMF guru and manufacturer of high intensity systems. Don't get me wrong, they do have their place, but it's generally focused more on horses and clinical treatments of acute cases managed by trained and licensed health professionals. More on this later.

Pulsed electromagnetic fields travel like waves, somewhat analogous to sound wave propagation. If we are talking about music, then the *intensity* would be comparable to the volume of the music. This amplitude is analogous to the amount of energy carried by the wave to induce a charge in the cells. *Therefore, the intensity of PEMF has a direct correlation to how much voltage is induced in the cells of the body.* So, in the above example if someone is telling you to buy as much intensity as you can afford, they are also saying to turn up the volume as loud as you can possibly stand or turn up the voltage to as much as your cells can tolerate.

Look at it this way. What happens when someone turns up the volume of any kind of music too loud? Eventually it's going to hurt your ears and possibly damage your hearing. You'll cover your ears to protect them. Your cells react the same way and close down to protect themselves if something too intense impacts them. This is just the opposite of what you want to happen. You want the cell membrane to open up, to resonate and allow more efficient absorption of nutrients along with the elimination of metabolic wastes. You don't want the cell to get in any kind of defensive mode that impacts or is disruptive to normal cellular functions.

It's also the same way with frequencies. If the cells in the body are impacted with very high frequencies, which are far above their own low frequencies, then this is disharmonious or dissonant to the cells. Several scientific studies have examined the effects of high-frequency electromagnetic fields (EMFs) on cellular functions. These studies indicate that high-frequency EMFs can impact biological systems in various ways, potentially disrupting cellular activities and leading to altered biological and mental functions.

1. **Cellular Stress Responses**: High-frequency EMFs can induce cellular stress responses, altering cell signaling pathways and gene expression. This can affect cell growth, differentiation and survival.

2. **Metabolic Disruptions**: Exposure to high-frequency EMFs has been shown to influence metabolic processes, potentially leading to oxidative stress and changes in cellular metabolism.

3. **Impact on Cell Membranes**: High-frequency EMFs can alter cell membrane permeability, affecting ion channels and the distribution of ions like calcium, which are crucial for various cellular processes.

Overall, the effects of high-frequency EMFs on cells depend on factors like the frequency, intensity and duration of exposure.

Resonance - The Key to Unlocking the Cell

Everything vibrates and has a frequency. It's is the nature of Nature in regard to all matter and energy… both of which are one and the same. Quantum field theory considers matter to be an excitation or a 'disturbance' in the electromagnetic field. Electromagnetism is one of the four fundamental forces of Nature. Yes, there may be a fifth force, but the jury is still out on this matter.

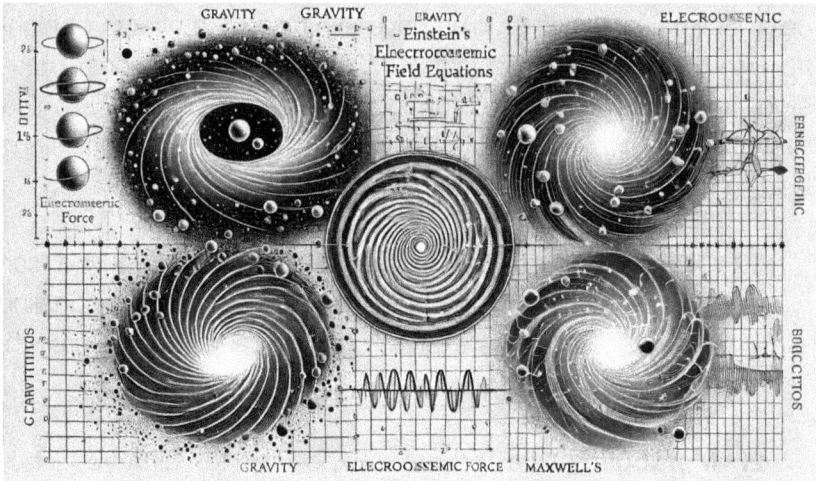

The four fundamental forces of nature are:

1 – Gravity

2 – Electromagnetic Force

3 – Weak Nuclear Force

4 – Strong Nuclear Force

In the realm of electromagnetic forces, resonance plays a crucial role in various phenomena, particularly in the context of electromagnetic waves. Understanding and manipulating PEMF resonance to tune in and harmonize with the bio-electromagnetic systems in the human body is essential to enhance efficient energy transfer, signal transmission and cellular communication.

The four forces are fundamental in the sense that they are believed to be the basic forces from which all other forces and energy derive. They play a crucial role in understanding the behavior of matter and energy in the universe. There is something intuitively grounding to know that PEMF is one of the fundamental forces of Nature that is used to improve health. In my opinion, it is one of the primary constituents of the 'spark of life.'

'The field is the sole governing agency of the particle' – Albert Einstein

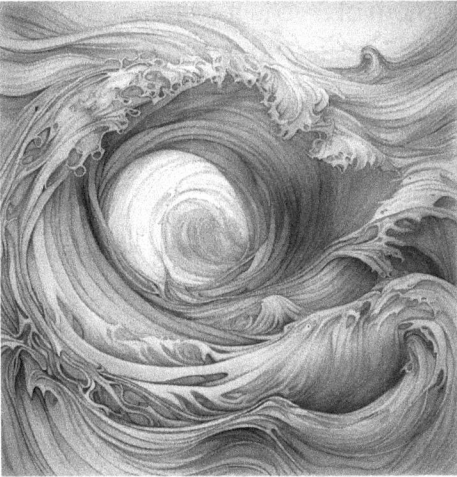

As stated earlier in the book, resonance in the body occurs *when the frequency and intensity of the stimulus is the same as the natural vibrational frequency of the cells.* When this happens, the cells respond positively and synchronize to the stimulus being presented. It's like the two tuning forks mentioned in Chapter 2. When tuning forks are placed in close proximity to each other, one tuning fork can *induce* the other to start vibrating through a phenomenon known as *sympathetic resonance*. This is exactly what needs to happen to the cells in the body.

Let's take it one step further with this analogy. What happens to speakers if you turn up the volume of music too much? The speakers, just like the cells in your body, can over modulate and become impaired or possibly become permanently damaged. We don't want to over modulate the cells. We want to harmonize or synchronize with them in *sympathy* by using resonating intensities at their corresponding natural voltage.

Intensity controls how much voltage is induced (more on this later). We want to induce resonating currents of the same voltage to charge the cells. The higher the intensity… the more current or voltage is induced within the cells. With high intensity systems the induced current is strong enough to contract muscles to varying degrees depending on how high the PEMF device is set. With low intensity systems, most people don't feel anything. This is a good sign. It takes on average a minimum of 3 volts to contract a muscle in the body. Now let's look at this in a little more detail.

Cell Voltage

Healthy cells have an average voltage of 25 mV (millivolts). Note: *You will also see in the literature where cellular voltage is quoted to be 70 to 90 mV (millivolts).* The first voltage mentioned (25 mV) is the voltage measured directly on the body (in vivo) versus cells measured in a petri dish (70 to 90 mV) in a laboratory (in vitro). For the purpose of this example, we shall use 25 millivolts (mV) going forward.

25 mV is a very low voltage. To put this voltage into perspective, 25 millivolts is 25/1000th of 1 volt or .025 volts. This is _60 times less_ than the voltage of an AA battery. If you wet your thumb and index finger and press them against each end of an AA battery, you won't feel a thing. Absolutely nothing. So, reduce that by 60 times to match or resonate with the cells' actual voltage in the body. To resonate with the cells' voltage, you *shouldn't* be feeling anything

during a PEMF treatment. Note: Sometimes, some people do feel a subtle or slight tingling, but very little else. Of course, I'm speaking about using low intensity PEMF in this case.

As stated before, the minimum voltage needed to induce muscles to contract is approximately 3 volts. This is over *120 times* more than the average voltage of a cell in the body. Some high-intensity systems go far beyond this level of voltage by thousands of times. In my opinion once again, it's all about creating resonance and coherence with the cells to *vibrate and resonate in sympathy* with them. Synchronize with their inherent low voltage. Don't shock them or hit them with a big electric spike that puts them in a defensive or protective mode. I believe this shock approach numbs the neural pain receptors and is not as conducive to healing although it can block or mask pain.

Let's look at this again with another analogy. When you charge a battery, you need to match or resonate with the actual voltage of the battery. You wouldn't charge a 12-volt car battery with 720 volts (60 times more) or with 1440 volts (120 times more). Same as with PEMF therapy if your beliefs are aligned with the natural, resonating theory of therapeutic health.

If you can feel the charge like you can with high intensity systems, then the charge is not resonating with the cells' actual voltage. Instead, it is OVER charging the cells (more is better approach). It's early days in the world of treating people with PEMF, therefore no one knows the long-term effects of high intensity PEMF. Yes, it delivers some beneficial results like knocking out pain very quickly. Most rapid changes in the body are often linked to a masking effect rather than genuine healing. True healing requires time.

It's also interesting to analyze intensity relative to the Earth's magnetic field strength and do some comparisons. Depending on your latitude, the earth's natural magnetic field intensity ranges from approximately 0.65 gauss nearing the North or South Poles going down to 0.25 gauss at the equator. For the example below, I will use an intensity of 0.40 gauss. A gauss is a unit of measurement for the strength of a static (constantly on) electromagnetic field.

I had a high intensity PEMF system that could produce 24,000 gauss. I know of at least one high intensity system that can generate up to 40,000 gauss. MRI medical scanners generate electromagnetic intensities ranging between 2,000 and 70,000 gauss. 2,000 gauss is 5,000 times stronger than the earth's natural magnetic field strength. 70,000 gauss would be 175,000 times stronger.

When you have an MRI scan, *everyone else gets out of the room.* The technicians are also protected by electromagnetic shields that are built into the walls, floors and ceilings of the entire room where the MRI scanner resides. This should serve as some kind of warning signpost for anyone considering a high intensity PEMF treatment or purchasing a high intensity system. Just as important, I wonder about the effects of long-term exposure to individual therapist applying high intensity systems on people and horses daily. I know the people treating horses have to be in the electromagnetic field with some high intensity applicator systems.

As stated previously, high intensity systems may have their place, especially for acute injuries, but it should only be administered by a trained health professional. It's also something I would not recommend doing on a daily basis. Personally, looking at the research, I wouldn't get close to fields of that strength. I *do* recommend low intensity PEMF on a daily basis if you can afford to invest in one for you and your family. I recommend a daily dose to keep cellular voltage up to a higher average threshold, which helps to maintain a higher overall cellular efficiency. If a cellular charge last approximately six hours on average, it would be best to have a PEMF treatment once or twice a day. It's very analogous to charging your smart phone. Again, that's if you own a PEMF system.

Law of Reciprocity

If I can see you, then you can see me.

If I can hear you, then you can hear me.

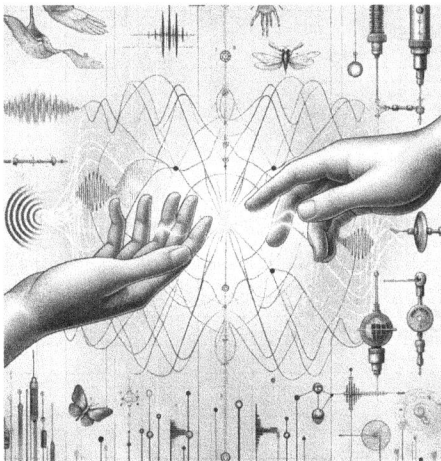

An important element in energy medicine is the law of reciprocity or the biological reciprocity principle. The nature of this principle, which is operational within the body and also within Nature, reflects how fundamental communication works on many different levels. By communication in this sense, I mean the transmission and reception of information or bioelectrical energy that enhances or maintains balance or a stable state of equilibrium in the body.

The law of reciprocity states that the frequency and bioelectrical potential a healthy cell *emits* is the same frequency and bioelectrical potential (voltage) that is readily *absorbed* by the cell. Like attracts like. This principle of reciprocity applies to how cells respond to electromagnetic signals. Matching frequency and the bioelectrical potential or voltage of cells can elicit a favorable physiological response. This response can be seen as increased cellular activity, improved metabolic efficiency, activation of signaling pathways or modulation of gene expression. It can also influence various cellular processes, including transmembrane potential changes, ion channel activity and downstream signaling events.

A common example is a TV antenna. When an antenna is tuned to a specific frequency, it is most effective at receiving signals of that very same frequency. This tuning is achieved by adjusting the antenna design to match the wavelength of the desired signal. When a signal of the resonating frequency is received, the antenna responds to the resonate frequency, amplifying the signal for further processing. The antenna is also automatically and reciprocally tuned to transmit the same frequencies it's designed to receive.

Similarly, in cellular reciprocity with bioelectrical signals, cells may be thought of as "tuned" to specific frequencies and voltages due to their biochemical activities and intrinsic electromagnetic properties. When a signal matches the resonant frequency and cellular voltage of a cell, it is more likely to elicit a strong and favorable positive response in the cell.

In summary, the analogy between cellular reciprocity and the tuned antenna illustrates how resonance phenomena are fundamental to both cellular biology and electromagnetic communication systems, highlighting the interconnectedness of biological and electromagnetic principles.

Research Studies

Most clinical research on PEMF therapy is conducted using low-intensity PEMF. I've read just the opposite on several websites selling high intensity systems. That's just not true at all. If you have the time, you can go to PubMed or other medical study databases and search for PEMF studies and wade through the literature like I have done. The lion's share is low intensity for the following reasons:

Safety considerations: Low-intensity PEMF waveforms are considered safer for human use by researchers. High-intensity waveforms can potentially cause adverse effects such as excessive nerve stimulation, severe muscle contractions and other discomforts. By using low-intensity waveforms, researchers aim to minimize the risk of any adverse reactions or harm to participants for liability reasons.

Compliance and acceptance: Low-intensity waveforms are more likely to be tolerated by individuals, increasing compliance with the treatment protocol. Higher intensity waveforms may cause discomfort or lead to a greater perception of the treatment as invasive, potentially reducing patient acceptance, adherence to the therapy and patients withdrawing from the study.

Efficacy exploration: Research in the field of PEMF therapy is still evolving, and there is ongoing debate about the optimal parameters for maximum efficacy. Many studies focus on determining the therapeutic effects of low-intensity waveforms to establish a baseline and understand the potential benefits of PEMF therapy. Once the effects of low-intensity waveforms are better understood, researchers can further investigate higher intensity waveforms and their potential applications.

Biological Windows – Proof that Less is More

"Small is Powerful, Less is More."
- Dr. Ross Adey

In the mid-1960s, Dr Ross Adey, who was an Australian-born professor of anatomy and physiology at the UCLA School of Medicine came up with the term "biological window" It has also been called the Adey Window. The Adey window describes the narrow parameters under which a very weak and non-thermal electromagnetic signal has a positive and resonating physiological effect on a human cell.

The biological window of resonance is a range of frequencies and intensities and that are readily accepted by the body and converted to positive physiological responses. Adey found that there exists a narrow range (sweet spot) of electromagnetic frequencies, typically between 0.1 to 50 Hertz, in which cells and tissues exhibit heightened sensitivity and response to external electromagnetic signals. This sensitivity is due to resonance effects and the ability of these frequencies to influence cellular processes including improved ion transport and cell signaling.

Signals that fall outside the biological window have little or no effect. In some cases, there can be negative or toxic effects if the frequencies or intensities are too high. As an analogy, sound can be very pleasant when listening to your favorite music. On the other hand, sound can be destructive like the sound of an explosion, which can permanently damage hearing. These findings have led to investigations into the potential therapeutic applications in various medical contexts, such as promoting tissue repair, bone healing and the treatment for certain neurological conditions.

Research has shown that living tissues readily detect, absorb and utilize electromagnetic signals within some frequency ranges and completely ignore other frequencies naturally encountered in the frequency spectrum. This is the Law of Reciprocity at work.

To measure the physiological effect, Adey observed the calcium output of a rabbit's brain cells. He showed that this effect could only be triggered using very low magnetic field intensities and a low frequency (16 Hz). Starting up at super-low intensities, there was no positive reaction until the intensity reached a certain level within a narrow range. Once the intensity got over a certain level, the cell shut down and became unresponsive.

Since Dr Adey's initial research, the medical literature has shown strong scientific consensus that a *biological window of resonance* exists and is a very important factor in delivering PEMF treatments for a positive cellular response. Less is more when it comes to PEMF intensity and there's also the frequency, which was also low (16 Hz) in this study.

Safety of PEMF

The ICNIRP (International Commission on Non-Ionizing Radiation Protection) is an *independent* non-profit organization that provides scientific advice and guidance on the health and environmental effects of non-ionizing radiation (NIR) to protect people and the environment from detrimental NIR exposure. Non-ionizing radiation is a type of radiation that doesn't have enough energy to change the structure of atoms or molecules in the cells. In other words, this means it can't cause damage to your body's cells and DNA.

A PEMF device needs to be able to resonate with the cells in problem areas of the body but yet be safe enough to be in compliance to the safety standards. **The DIN 0848 safety standard for time varying waves (PEMFs) states that the intensity should never exceed 400 µT or 4 gauss.**

Reference levels of exposure to time varying electric fields

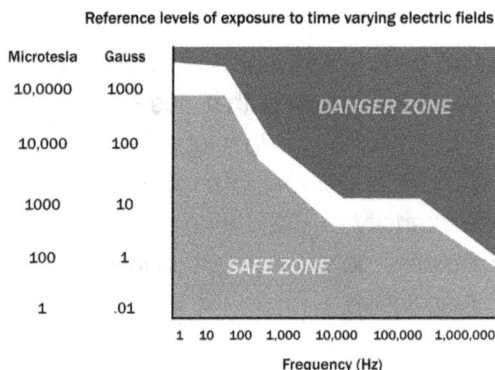

The ICNIRP is a global authority on safety related to electromagnetic energy. The European Union, the FDA and the TGA in Australia rely on their findings. According to the ICNIRP, the limiting values for safety of time varying PEMF are dependent on both the frequency (measured in Hz) and the flux density, which is measured in microtesla (µT). Magnetic flux density is a measure of the strength of a magnetic field over a specific area. It quantifies how much magnetic flux passes through a given area, reflecting the concentration or intensity of the magnetic field at that location

By safe, this means that the cells and tissues are not exposed to ionizing radiation that can cause burns, radiation sickness, mutation, cancer or genetic damage. The higher the applied frequency the lower the limit value for intensity that is safe. This means, if you apply a very low frequency (within the earth frequency range of 1-50 Hz) you can apply somewhat higher intensities.

Safety concerns surrounding high intensity PEMF have been addressed by the International Commission on Non-Ionizing Radiation Protection (ICNIRP), which has established guidelines for safe EMF exposure. These recommendations have raised questions and concerns about the safety of many high intensity PEMF devices currently on the market.

Critical Point

The limited value according to the ICNIRP for low frequency, time varying electromagnetic waves in the range from 0 to 25 HZ is 5000 microtesla (μT) or 50 gauss. One high intensity PEMF device can generate magnetic fields up to 9,360 gauss. There are other high intensity systems on the market that are over double that value.

If the frequency is over 25 Hz, the limiting value for safety is only 5 microtesla (μT) or .05 gauss! It means, that the ICNIRP assumes, that time varying PEMF over 25 HZ with a higher intensity than 5 microtesla (μT) or .05 gauss may potentially cause cell damage.

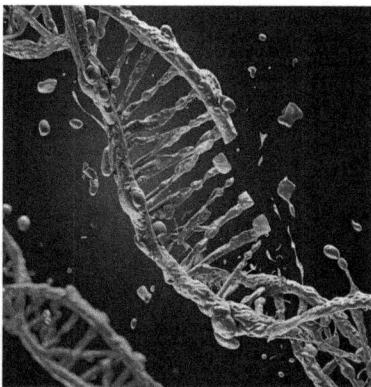

There is a clinical study on PubMed, [Extremely low-frequency electromagnetic fields cause DNA strand breaks in normal cells], which has shown that the DNA in cells fragment or split apart with a frequency of 100 Hz and an intensity of 56 gauss for a duration of 45 minutes. The study showed that 100 Hz and

5.6 mT (56 gauss) had a genotoxic effect on the cells. Genotoxic refers to agents or substances that damage the genetic information within a cell, which can cause genetic mutations, chromosomal fragmentation, cancer or errors in DNA replication and repair. There are other studies showing cell fragmentation on PubMed, so this is not a single or isolated study. There are also conflicting studies showing just the opposite.

It's essential to look beyond marketing claims you read on the internet from manufacturers or distributors of PEMF systems and focus on scientific evidence and safety guidelines when considering PEMF therapy. Low intensity devices, operating at levels close to the Earth's natural magnetic field strength, have far more extensive research supporting their efficacy and safety across a wide range of health conditions. There are far less clinical studies on high intensity PEMFs.

There are also no long-term studies of PEMF comparing the use of high intensity systems versus low intensity on people. For me, it's very difficult to go past the safety guidelines of the International Commission on Non-Ionizing Radiation Protection (ICNIRP), especially when you look at the tissue culture study I noted above.

In my opinion, it all comes down to common sense and some gut intuition. Do you want to get treated with naturally occurring frequencies and intensities the same as the earth's; or do you want to expose yourself to levels thousands of times stronger?

I have raised my concerns about the potential for DNA fragmentation when cells are exposed to electromagnetic fields above certain intensities. You can find studies showing DNA fragmentation on many different levels of intensity. There are also studies indicating that low-frequency electromagnetic fields at relatively low intensities may induce DNA strand breaks in cells. Other studies show no breakage at much higher levels, so there's no clear level or threshold to be found where cellular fragmentation may occur or not occur. Many other factors such as pulse duration, frequency, waveform, flux density and exposure time play crucial roles in the biological effects of PEMF therapy. Many of the studies are cells cultured in a petri dish, which is nothing like the environment in the body. Also, many studies give very little detail on all of the parameters used in the study.

All of this raises a discrepancy with the International Commission on Non-Ionizing Radiation Protection (ICNIRP) guidelines, which recommend exposure limits of approximately 50 gauss (5,000 microtesla) for frequencies up to 25 Hz to ensure safety from non-ionizing radiation. The fact that many therapeutic PEMF devices exceed these limits suggests a need to reconcile these differences. Medical devices are designed with safety protocols and are regulated by agencies like the FDA, which consider the benefits versus potential risks. From its past history, anything the FDA approves in my opinion should be carefully scrutinized. The majority of PEMF devices on the market are not regulated or officially approved as a medical device.

Another significant concern is that PEMF therapy is frequently administered by individuals who are not licensed health professionals and often lack comprehensive medical training. This lack of expertise can lead to improper use of equipment, incorrect settings and failure to recognize contraindications or adverse effects, thereby increasing the risk to patients. The importance of professional training, regulatory oversight and adherence to safety guidelines is sorely lacking in most countries.

Devices like Repetitive Transcranial Magnetic Stimulation (rTMS) operate at intensities of 10,000 to 20,000 gauss, yet clinical evidence supports their safety when used according to established protocols. Doctors, specifically psychiatrists, also do electroconvulsive shock therapy (ECT) where they shock the brain with voltage ranges from 70 to 450 volts. 450 volts would be over 6,000 times stronger than the cellular voltage of the brain cells. I assume they say this is safe too. What do you think?

In conclusion, while high-intensity PEMF devices are used therapeutically and are said to be safe when properly applied, there is a discrepancy between recommended exposure limits and actual practice. The administration of PEMF therapy by unlicensed individuals further underscores the need for regulatory oversight, proper training and strict adherence to safety guidelines to ensure patient well-being and maximize therapeutic benefits.

CHAPTER 8
Purchasing a PEMF System

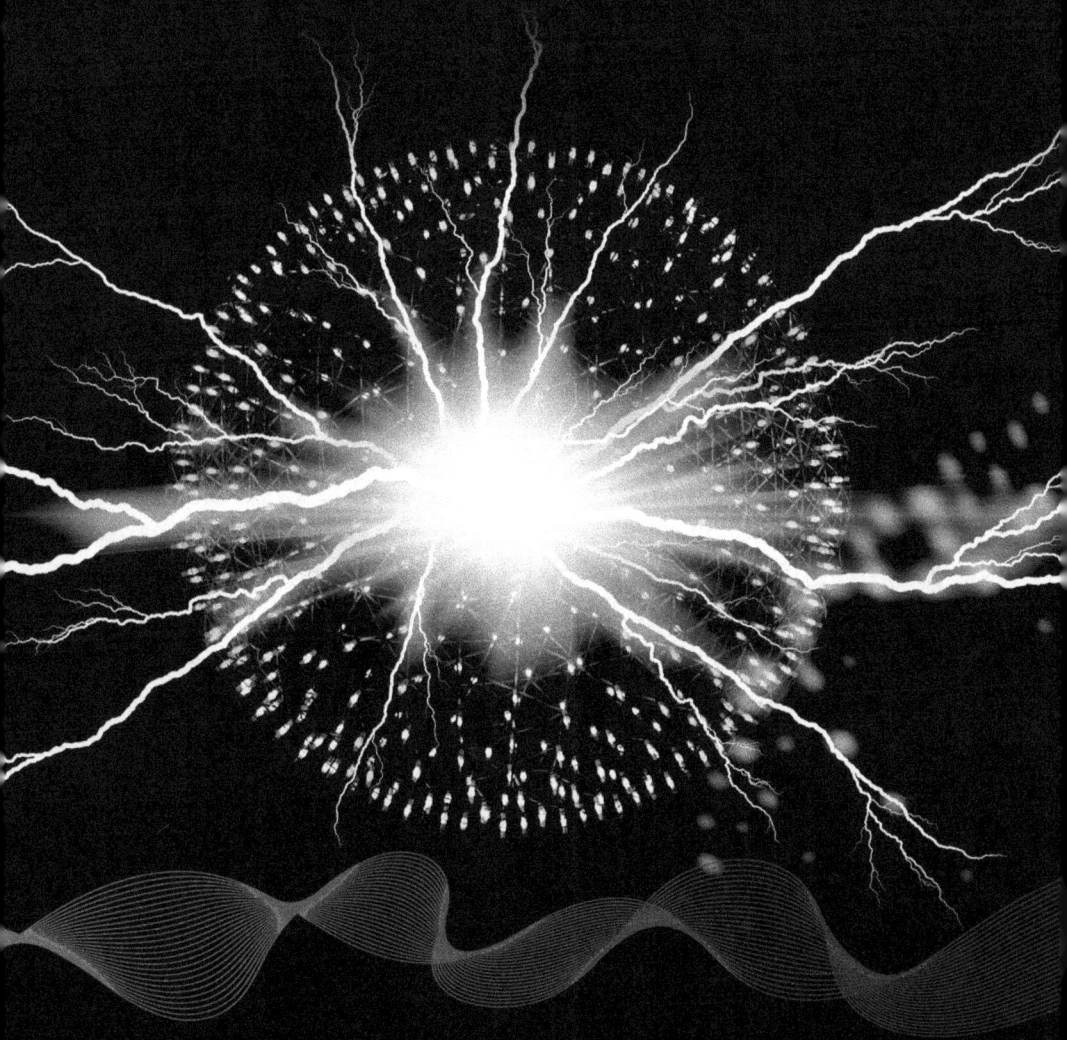

CHAPTER 8

Purchasing a PEMF System

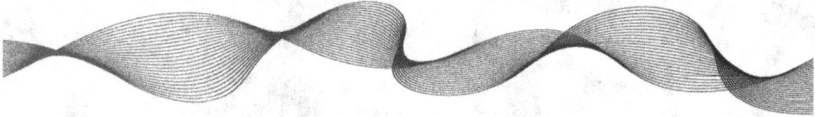

Choosing a PEMF System

I trust my personal bias and preference for low intensity systems is fairly evident by this point in the book. When I first started looking into PEMF years ago, I didn't have any bias, but eventually followed my instinct to keep aligned with nature and the natural forces of the earth along with incorporating the principles of resonance, coherence and the law of reciprocity.

There are many kinds of PEMF systems out on the market and this makes if very confusing when you first start looking around. Some manufacturers of PEMF systems have been around for nearly thirty years, while others are relatively new to the market. PEMF was basically born in Germany in the mid-eighties. This is where PEMF initially appeared in the marketplace, at least for the general public. One of the companies that grew out of this is the manufacturer of the system I presently use. It's very important to look at the history of the company you purchase from and to stay away from cheap systems that purport to do so many different things all in one system such as PEMF, far infrared, red-light therapy, negative ions, natural crystals, magnetic layers and so on.

Besides the high versus low intensity types of systems to choose from, one also has to consider smaller localized PEMF devices. These devices can be battery powered or AC from household power. They are designed for targeting specific areas of the body, and if battery powered, are also designed for portability. They definitely have their place for personal use if they are up to the quality level of Micro-Pulse.

For overall health care and getting the best of both worlds, I suggest a PEMF system that has at least three different applicators (applicators are where the PEMF is emitted - sort of like speakers). I suggest a full-body mat and one or two smaller applicators for more targeted use. You may lose portability with a bigger system, but overall, I feel it's very important to treat the whole body all at once. Ideally you have both types of systems if you require portability.

I'll take you through my decision-making process when purchasing my first system. Here are my reasons for choosing this system. You can find out more about the systems from the QR codes.

I use a low intensity system for myself and the people I treat. I feel the present system I use is one of the best for many reasons. You can find out more about the systems on the websites: www.pemf.com.au or www.pemfinc.com or have a look in the resource section of the book.

I chose the system for the following reasons:

1 – The system has been manufactured in Germany since 1995. The systems have been upgraded seven times over the years and they are continually working on new innovations. At present, they are the only company in the world with a fully integrated brain entrainment and biofeedback system, which are offered as optional accessories.

2 – The system utilizes two of the most efficient waveforms (triple sawtooth and square wave) for superior voltage induction in the cells. This has increased the resonance potential for people who positively respond to one waveform over the other or the combination of the two together. It's a very important feature that increases the probability of seeing more positive results.

3 – Several of the systems can simultaneously run two different applicators (mat, pad or spot) at full power. This is a great time saver for a user and/or practitioner to be able to treat two different localized areas of the body at the same time.

4 – Some of the systems have far infrared built into the full-body mat. The far infrared is nothing like a sauna experience. Just hop on the mat with any type of clothing. There's no perfuse sweating or showering required. The most common thing I hear from people is that they don't want to get up and leave their cozy warm nest on the mat.

5 – One of the one touch automated programs creates the Solfeggio frequencies in electromagnetic waves. The Solfeggio frequencies are a set of musical tones that have origins dating back to medieval Western Christianity and Eastern Indian religions. The concept of the Solfeggio frequencies gained renewed interest in the 20th

century, particularly in the fields of sound healing and alternative medicine. Some proponents claim that these specific frequencies have healing properties and can bring about various therapeutic effects when used in music or sound therapy.

6 – Some of the systems have an integrated settings guide. This is a feature that lists approximately 300 different health conditions with recommended treatment settings to use for each of the three applicators.

7 – The systems are low intensity and low frequency systems that align with the frequencies and intensities of the earth and Nature. This is more of a natural way to healing. What's most important is that it works and is also very safe.

8 – The systems are globally certified medical devices. All of their systems comply with all present global electrical certification standards, which many other PEMF systems fail to meet.

It's important to note that the choice between low and high-intensity PEMF systems may depend on individual needs, health conditions and budget, to name a few. Consulting with an experienced healthcare professional in the PEMF field before purchasing and using any PEMF device is recommended to ensure it aligns with your specific health goals and requirements.

Cheap & Counterfeit PEMF Devices

Sometimes I'm asked why the systems I sell are so expensive compared to others on the market. It's a common question and a very good one. The models of PEMF machines that I use are actually priced in the middle range compared to the whole spectrum of systems available in the market for home or professional use.

In the global market place, there are small portable units of various descriptions starting from several hundred dollars, up to systems that can cost over a hundred thousand dollars. The most expensive PEMF systems tend to be high intensity systems, which I advise people wanting to use PEMF on a daily basis to avoid. Unfortunately, with the rise in popularity of PEMF, there has been a surge in the market of cheap imitations and counterfeits, particularly from China. I'm trying to shed some light on why it's crucial to avoid these imitations and how to identify and choose a quality PEMF system.

I point out to people all the time to avoid the lower end of the scale in regard to the cheap PEMF whole body systems. As mentioned earlier, be very careful with the systems that offer a full-body mat that purports to do a little bit of everything. I'm talking about mats that can range from USD $300 to USD $2,000 with one or more of the following features: PEMF, far infrared, negative ions, photon / red light therapy, crystals, natural gemstones, functional layering and certified semiprecious stones. They make it look like you are getting a little bit of everything for a great price. That's far from the case once you look into it further. And, there's always the fact that you do get what you pay for.

1. Cost

Regarding the proverbial bottom line, you can go to Alibaba online and purchase the exact same systems directly from the Chinese manufacturer for three to four times less than an advertised retail price. The only difference is that they won't have the company branding on it. Literally, you can purchase a system that normally sells online for a retail price of USD $2,000 for around USD $250 plus shipping.

You can also find review websites with wonderful testimonials and high ratings for these systems, but they're just part of the 'marketing' by the manufacturers or distributors. Fake consumer review websites are prolific these days. Just like anything that's doing some good out there, which genuine PEMF does, there are those who want to cash in and take advantage of vulnerable people. People with chronic or serious health issues can be very vulnerable and susceptible to false or misleading advertising with what are simply counterfeit products with an attractive price. Buyer beware!

2. PEMF Output

When the questionable mats were dissected and cut open, it was found that they had a number of cheap AM radio ferrite rod coils. This was verified by an experienced professional with measuring equipment such as an oscilloscope and frequency spectrum analyzer. Here are a few reasons why an AM radio ferrite rod coil is not suitable for PEMF therapy:

1. Limited Frequency Range: AM radio ferrite rod coils are designed for radio frequencies in the kilohertz range, which is a much higher frequency range and not even close to the resonant low frequencies of the body. I kilohertz equals 1,000 hertz but AM radio frequencies can range from 530,000 Hz up to 1.7 million hertz. Genuine PEMF systems operate at much lower frequencies. Therefore, the therapeutic effects associated with low frequencies are likely to not be achievable using a high AM frequency radio coils, which weren't initially designed for PEMF systems.

2. Uncontrolled Magnetic Field: AM radio coils are not optimized for generating controlled and therapeutic magnetic fields. PEMF devices use specific coil designs (flat copper coils) and configurations to produce magnetic fields with controlled intensity and inductive waveforms.

3. Safety Concerns: Without proper design and control, using a ferrite rod coil may lead to uncontrolled electromagnetic fields, potentially causing safety concerns or unintended side effects.

The second thing that was found is that there is no signal generator, which is needed to generate and control specific waveforms in genuine PEMF systems. All the cheap systems do to generate their so-called PEMF, is to pulse on and off the 50 hertz or 60 hertz household mains power frequency, which is essentially dirty electricity. Bottom line, you are not getting anything close to therapeutic electromagnetic waves. You are also exposing yourself to dirty electricity and high radio frequencies.

Far Infrared

The cheap mats actually do produce heat, but it's basically an expense electric blanket, which again, is using dirty electricity to generate the heat.

Red Light Therapy

When the photon or red-light therapy outputs are precisely measured on the cheap systems, the radiance or strength of the red light output is so low that it's equivalent or no better than Christmas tree LED lights. These lights are approximately ten times below the minimum recommended level for red-light therapy to achieve therapeutic effects. Plus, the density or how close the lights are spaced together is very sparse. Quality red-light panels can have up to hundreds of LED lights. A genuine red-light panel of comparable size to the size of one of the cheap mats can have 500 to 600 LED lights radiating far more therapeutic light. The fake mats have around 30 to 60 LED lights generating ordinary red light. Get the picture?

Negative Ions

These fake systems do not generate much or any negative ions at all. It will cost $50 to $100 on Amazon, but you can purchase a Negative Ion Testing Test Meter and test it yourself.

Bottom Line

We all know this; you really do get what you pay for with PEMF systems along with most everything else. If you find a PEMF system with a list of features and functionalities that is far cheaper than other long established PEMF systems that have been proven in the market place and stand the test of time, then buyer beware. With these kind of systems, you're not getting much or very little beneficial PEMFs. Bottom line, you can also purchase these systems direct from the manufacturer on Alibaba for three to four times less than they are being offered at retail if you have to have one.

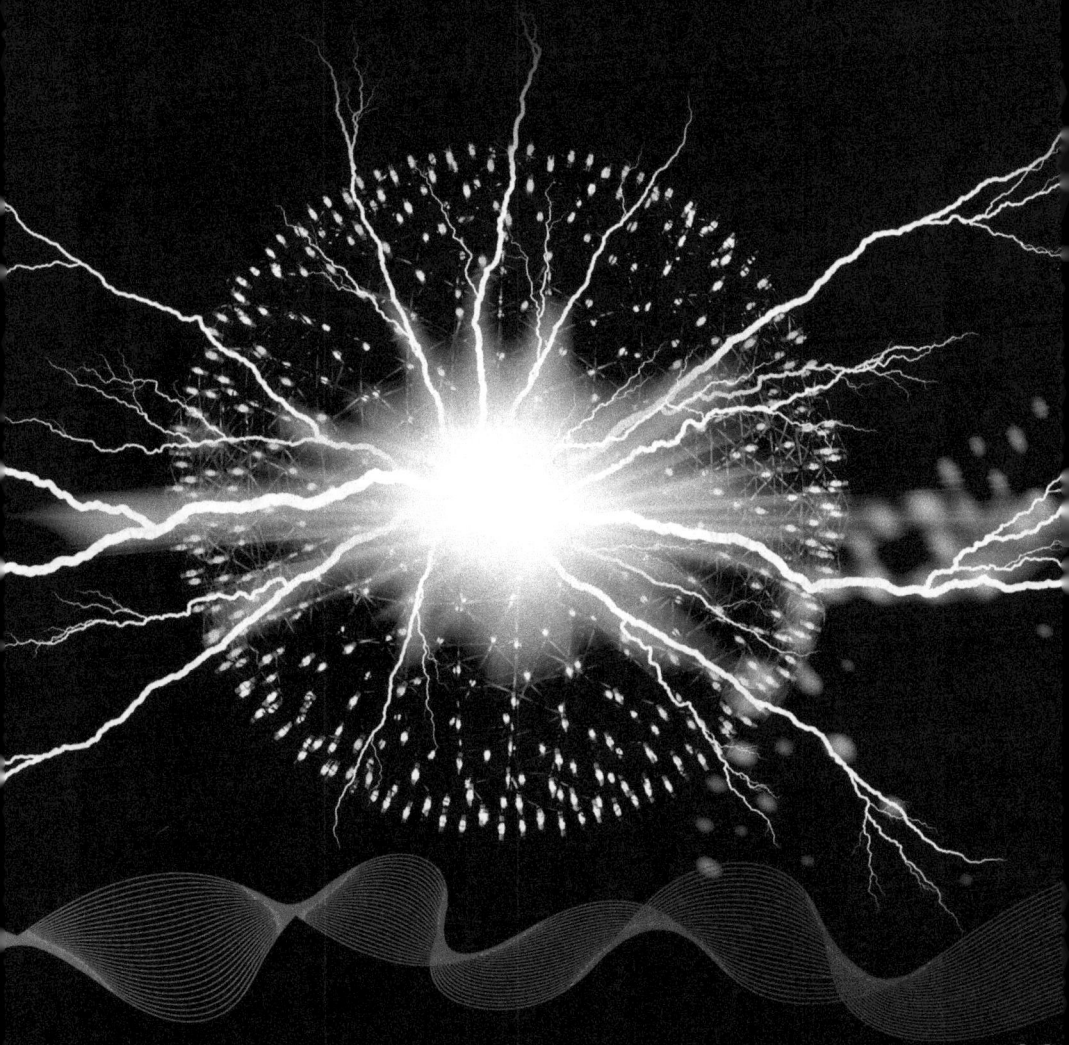

CHAPTER 9
Resources

CHAPTER 9

Resources

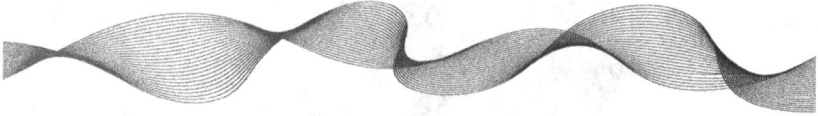

Books on PEMF

There are many books on PEMF Therapy, so I suggest doing a search on Amazon or Google.

Here's a list of books and authors on PEMF therapy:

1. "The Practice of Magnetic Field Therapy" by Dr. Christian Thuile, M.D. published in English in 2000. The first good book on PEMF written by a practicing doctor in Germany.

2. "Recharging Your Life" by Gary Woolums published by Global Publishing Group.

3. "PEMF - The Fifth Element of Health: Learn Why Pulsed Electromagnetic Field (PEMF) Therapy Supercharges Your Health Like Nothing Else!" by Bryant A. Meyers One of my favorites and highly recommended.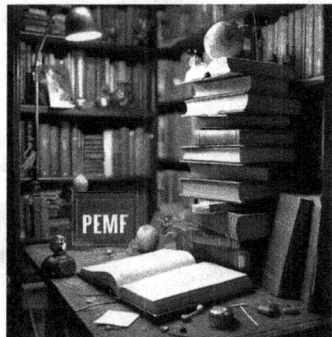

4. "The Body Electric: Electromagnetism and the Foundation of Life" by Robert O. Becker and Gary Selden - Although not specifically about PEMF therapy, this classic book explores the role of electromagnetism in biological systems and its implications for health and healing. Difficult read and very technical.

5. Energy Medicine: The Scientific Basis by Dr. James L Oschman PhD. The seminal work on the biophysics of the human body.

6. "Frequency Specific Microcurrent in Pain Management" by Carolyn McMakin - Although not specifically about PEMF therapy, this book discusses the use of microcurrent therapy, which shares some similarities with PEMF therapy for managing pain and promoting healing.

7. "The Resonance Effect: How Frequency Specific Microcurrent Is Changing Medicine" by Carolyn McMakin - Another book that explores the therapeutic potential of frequency-specific microcurrent therapy, which has overlapping applications with PEMF therapy.

8. "Healing is Voltage: The Handbook" by Jerry L. Tennant - While not exclusively focused on PEMF therapy, this book discusses the importance of electrical voltage in the body's healing processes and explores various modalities, which include PEMF therapy for restoring balance.

9. "The Field: The Quest for the Secret Force of the Universe" by Lynne McTaggart - While not specifically about PEMF therapy, this book explores the concept of the "field" and its potential role in healing and consciousness.

10. "We Are Electric: Inside the 200-Year Hunt for Our Body's Bioelectric Code and What the Future Holds" by Sally Adee - Science journalist Sally Adee breaks open the field of bioelectricity, the electric currents that run through our bodies and every living thing. Highly recommend it.

11. "Power Tools for Health: How Pulsed Magnetic Fields (PEMFs) Help You" by M. Sara Rosenthal & Dr. William Pawluk- This book provides an overview of PEMF therapy and its potential health benefits, as well as practical guidance on using PEMF devices. It is high intensity biased.

12. "Electric Body, Electric Health: Using the Electromagnetism Within (and Around) You to Rewire, Recharge and Raise Your Voltage" by Eileen Day McKusick. This book looks at our bodies and teaches people how to raise their voltage.

List of Resources

1. Scientific Journals and Research Articles:

- Journal of Clinical Orthopedics and Trauma
- Bio Electro Magnetics
- Journal of Alternative and Complementary Medicine
- PLOS One
- Journal of Electromagnetic Waves and Applications
- IEEE Transactions on Biomedical Engineering
- Journal of Electromagnetic Biology and Medicine
- Electromagnetic Biology and Medicine

2. Professional Organizations and Associations:

- International Society for Electromagnetic Medicine (ISEM) - Website: https://isem.org/

- BioElectroMagnetics Society (BEMS) - Website: https://www.bems.org/

- European BioElectroMagnetics Association (EBEA) - Website: https://ebea.org/

- International Society for BioElectroMagnetism (ISBEM) - Website: https://www.isbem.org/

- International Society for Electromagnetic Therapy (ISEMET)

- National Institutes of Health (NIH) - Electromagnetic Fields Research

- Australasian BioElectroMagnetics Society (EBMS)

- Foundation for Alternative & Integrative Medicine https://www.nfam.org/

- International Society for the Study of Subtle Energies and Energy Medicine (ISSSEEM) https://uia.org/s/or/en/1100016471

- International Commission on Non-ionizing Radiation Protection (ICNIRP) https://www.icnirp.org/

3. Research Databases:

- PubMed is a free resource supporting the search and retrieval of biomedical and life sciences literature. The PubMed database contains more than 37 million citations and abstracts of biomedical literature Website: https://pubmed.ncbi.nlm.nih.gov/

- ResearchGate is a professional network of over 25 million researchers to share and discover research, build their networks and advance their careers. Based in Berlin, ResearchGate was founded in 2008. Its mission is to connect the world of science and make research open to all. It's free. Website: https://www.researchgate.net/

- World Health Organization International Clinical Trials Registry Platform (ICTRP) - Website: https://www.who.int/clinical-trials-registry-platform

- National Center for Complementary and Integrative Health (NCCIH)

- Academia is a free resource offering access to one third of the world's research papers https://www.academia.edu

4. Regulatory Agencies and Guidelines:

- Food and Drug Administration (FDA) - Website: https://www.fda.gov/ - regulations and guidelines on PEMF devices

- European Commission - regulations and guidelines on PEMF devices

- European Medicines Agency (EMA) - Website: https://www.ema.europa.eu/

- International Electrotechnical Commission (IEC) - Website: https://www.iec.ch/

- National Institute for Occupational Safety and Health (NIOSH) - Website: https://www.cdc.gov/niosh/

- ICNIRP (International Commission on Non-Ionizing Radiation Protection) - aims to protect people and the environment against adverse effects of non-ionizing radiation (NIR). https://www.icnirp.org/

- Health Canada - Consumer and Clinical Radiation Protection Bureau

- Australian Therapeutic Goods Administration (TGA)

5. Reputable online resources and databases:

- National Center for Complementary and Integrative Health (NCCIH)

- Cochrane Library

- EMF Portal (EMF-Portal.org)

PEMF System Suppliers

PEMF Therapy

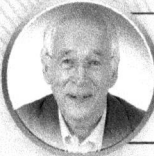

Free Consultations

Schedule an individual discussion to answer any questions about PEMF treatments, systems or training. Happy to have a chat.

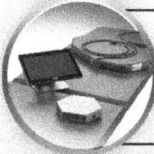

Purchase a PEMF System

Secure your health's future with our advanced PEMF systems. Receive complimentary expert guidance to inform and assist you in choosing the best solution for your special needs. Tailored treatment protocols provided with each system.

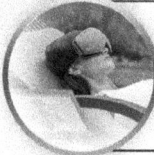

PEMF Therapy Training

Discover the benefits of PEMF therapy with our customized training program tailored to your personal needs. Acquire the skills to use PEMF in an existing health practice, gym, wellness center or starting a new business.

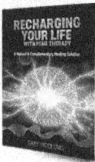

Read the New Book

Unlock the Secret Chapter!

Discover deeper insights and exclusive content with Recharging Your Life's secret chapter. This chapter delves into advanced techniques and personal anecdotes that are not included in the main content of the book.

How to Access the Secret Chapter:

1. **Scan the QR Code:** Use your smartphone camera or a QR code scanner app to scan the code below.
2. **Follow the Link:** The QR code will take you to a special webpage where you can read or download the secret chapter.
3. **Enjoy Exclusive Content:** Immerse yourself in the additional knowledge and stories that enhance your understanding of PEMF therapy.

**Visit www.pemfinc.com
to learn more to empower yourself with the best in
PEMF therapy!**

🌐 www.pemfinc.com 📞 516-473-0059 📍 Denver, USA

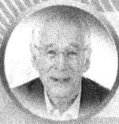

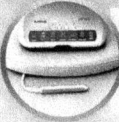

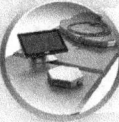

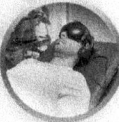

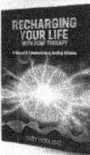

Molecular Hydrogen Inhalation

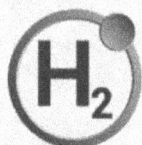

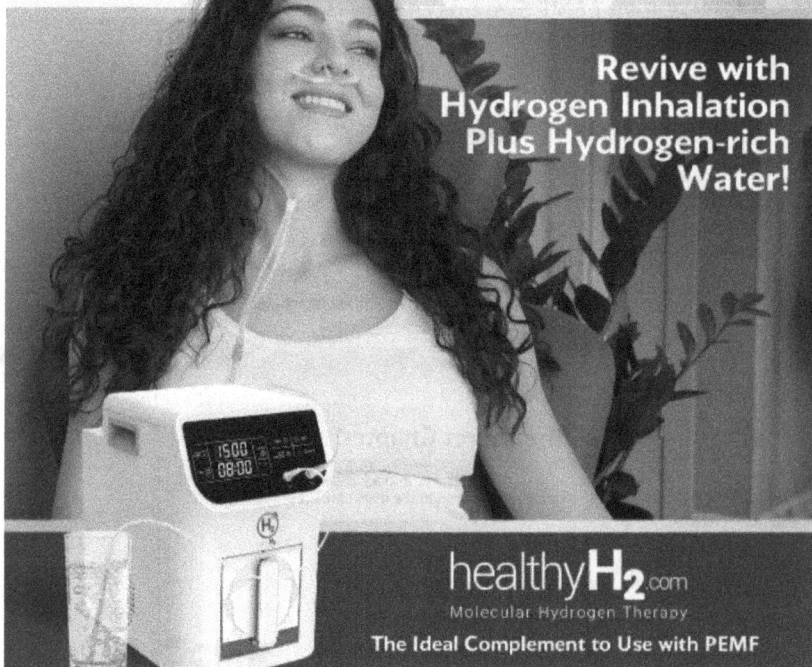

One Model for Every Need

- Backed by Clinical Research
- Proven Safe & Effective
- Just add Distilled Water
- Portable & Very Quiet

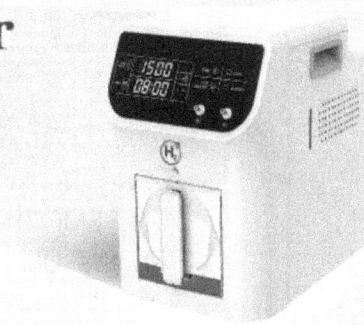

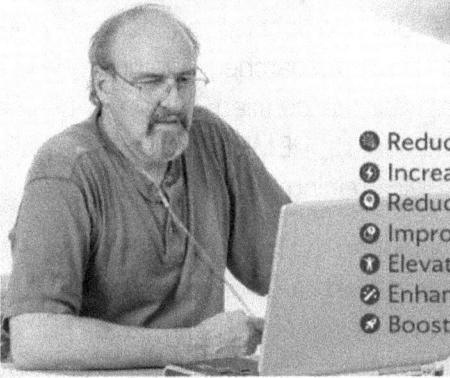

- Reduces Inflammation & Pain
- Increases Energy & Vitality
- Reduces Oxidative Stress
- Improves Cognitive Clarity
- Elevates Overall Well-being
- Enhances Nerve Repair
- Boosts Performance & Endurance

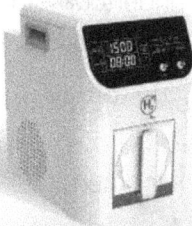

Features

- 300, 600, 900, 1200 & 1500 ml/min
- Brown's gas (H2+ O2)
- Timer: 1,2,3,5 & 8 hours
- SPE and PEM technology
- Water level detection monitor
- Total dissolved solids detection
- Hydrogen-rich water bubbler included

Non-toxic, non-invasive with no known side effects

Benefits shown in 1,200+ studies for 170 health conditions

www.healthyH2.com

177

AUTHOR PROFILE

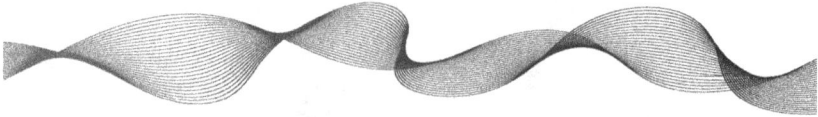

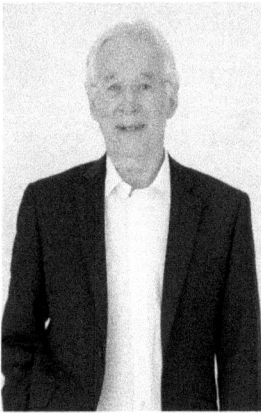

Gary Woolums is an author and the owner of PEMF Therapy Australia and PEMF Inc in the US. He is also an active PEMF practitioner, researcher, distributor and trainer. Gary is certified & trained by the Association of PEMF Professionals and the PEMF Training Academy in the US.

Gary attended the University of Iowa where he completed a four-year pre-medical program. He graduated cum laude with a Bachelor of Science degree in psychology then moved to San Francisco where he undertook studies for a master's degree in parapsychology and Eastern Studies.

Prior to discovering the healing benefits of PEMF technology, Gary also studied under a metaphysician and healer as part of his ongoing interest in health and personal development.

His early working life was spent in the energy industry doing research exploring alternative technologies to conserve energy. During the 80's, he started a successful solar energy company and a fundraising company. In 1991, after a severe back injury, Gary moved to Australia. He endured chronic pain for twenty-six years until he discovered the benefits of PEMF, which completely alleviated his back problem.

www.ingramcontent.com/pod-product-compliance
Lightning Source LLC
Chambersburg PA
CBHW072236270326
41930CB00010B/2146